Book 1: The BASICS

The **NUTRIENT** Diet

A Cognitive Behavioral Approach to Diet, Impulse Control, Habit Formation, Eating Behaviors & Weight Management

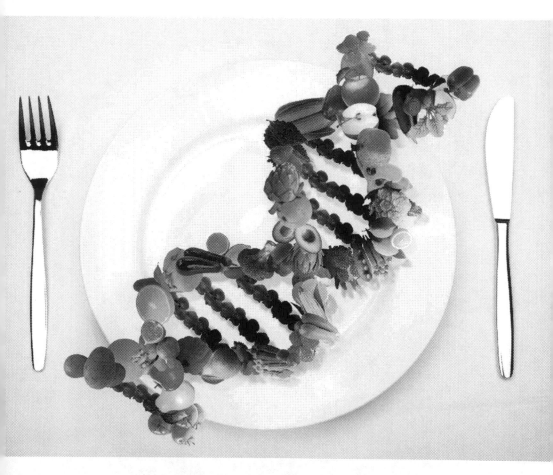

*Change Your Dietary Habits & Lifestyle Choices, **One Week** at a Time*

David A. Wright, MD, MM, MBA, MHSA (Dr. David)

Use *The Nutrient Diet* to help empower your lifestyle.

Use *The Nutrient Diet* to help inspire your daily habits.

Use *The Nutrient Diet* to help fuel your health and wellness choices.

Use *The Nutrient Diet* to help fuel your daily activities.

Use *The Nutrient Diet* to help ignite your ability to change the core of your body.

Use *The Nutrient Diet* to help energize your mind, body, spirit, and soul.

Use *The Nutrient Diet* to help you stay mentally refreshed and renewed.

The Nutrient Diet truly is nourishment for your mind, body, spirit, soul, and psyche.

Check us out online at www.mlcoga.com.

Book 1: The BASICS.

The **NUTRIENT** Diet

A Cognitive Behavioral Approach to Diet, Impulse Control,
Habit Formation, Eating Behaviors & Weight Management

Change Your Dietary Habits & Lifestyle Choices, One Week at a Time

David A. Wright, MD, MM, MBA, MHSA

With forewords by
Dr. Christopher M. Palmer (Harvard psychiatric expert on the ketogenic diet)
Dr. Todd M. Antin (Emory quadruple board-certified expert in psychiatry)
Revered Harlis R. Wright (pastor and former professor of science)

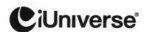

THE NUTRIENT DIET
A COGNITIVE BEHAVIORAL APPROACH TO DIET, IMPULSE
CONTROL, HABIT FORMATION, EATING BEHAVIORS & WEIGHT
MANAGEMENT

iUniverse books may be ordered through booksellers or by contacting:

iUniverse
1663 Liberty Drive
Bloomington, IN 47403
www.iuniverse.com
844-349-9409

ISBN: 978-1-6632-1017-3 (sc)
ISBN: 978-1-6632-1016-6 (e)

Library of Congress Control Number: 2021904712

Print information available on the last page.

iUniverse rev. date: 05/19/2021

About The NUTRIENT Diet

Since the 1980s I've literally observed hundreds of diet plans come and go—although, a few of them, like Weight Watchers ®, Jenny Craig ®, Slim Fast ® and Nutrisystem®, have appeared to stand the tests of time. However, most of them, seem to come and go like the wind. And, I got to see this up close and personal within my own family, within myself and within the clients of my practices. Through all of these observations, and taking an analytic approach to them both singularly and in aggregate, I came to the conclusion that the vast majority of diet plans and approaches "FAIL" because they expect the individual to make too many primary changes at once. In essence, they expect you to change overnight (instead of doing so gradually and naturally), leading most dieters feeling frustrated and overwhelmed. And, plans, goals and objectives tend to fail when they require too many steps too quickly. I base this opinion off of the "Simplicity Principle", which I state as 'the simpler something is to set up and begin, the more likely one is to consistently continue (i.e., perpetuate) it.' The reverse of that is the "Complexity Principle", which I state as 'the more complicated something is to set up, begin and/ or perpetuate, then the more likely one is to abruptly discontinue (i.e., abandon) it eventually.' The same is true of most diets (i.e., lifestyle modification plans [LMPs]). Because they are generally complex (and unpleasant), even when someone strives to make them easy, they are difficult to permanently install as a habit, routine &/or ritual. That's WHY it's so difficult for the vast majority of individuals to start, continue and complete a diet (or other lifestyle plan); and to continue to maintain the habits required to keep their new weight.

The Nutrient Diet is a completely new, bold, intelligent, modern, psychological approach to diet, health, wellness and weight management habits! The Nutrient Diet is a "Lifestyle Approach" for general & mental health based on sound psychological principles! The Nutrient Diet is 50% Diet and Nutrition, and 50% Cognitive and Behavioral Psychological Strategies for eating behaviors, dieting, impulse control and habit formation. The Nutrient Diet is the first book of its kind to take a "Cognitive Behavioral" (i.e., Psychological) approach to diet, nutrition, health, wellness, weight loss, weight management and lifestyle management! The Nutrient Diet truly is a "Trendsetter" in the diet, health, wellness, medicine, nutrition, weight loss, weight management and lifestyle fields! Not only does The Nutrient Diet show and explain WHAT you need to eat, The Nutrient Diet explains HOW & WHY you should eat it—based on sound, tested scientific data, clinical trials and psychological principles! The Nutrient Diet does so in a way that teaches and coaches you to make lifestyle changes easily, naturally, gradually and progressively so that you don't get frustrated and overwhelmed along the way... Even more, The Nutrient Diet augments other dietary plans (Like Nutrisystem ®, Weight Watchers ®, Slim Fast ® and Jenny Craig ®) with nutritional facts, concepts, principles and explanations in a straightforward way that makes it much less likely that you'll fail or abandon them. So, The Nutrient Diet will help you even if you're already using another dietary plan! The Nutrient Diet plays well with others! The Nutrient Diet is a must read for anyone interested in creating and maintaining good health and managing their weight without dreading it!

David A. Wright, MD, MM, MBA, MHSA (Dr. David)

Dr. Wright's new lifestyle, health, wellness, weight loss, nutrition & diet book, The Nutrient Diet, could not have come at a better time in history. Nutrition and diet are the building blocks of all metabolic activity, and they form the underpinnings of both general and mental health. I have been using ketogenic diets to treat patients with psychiatric disorders ranging from major depressive disorder to bipolar disorder to schizophrenia for almost two decades. As such, I understand all too well just how crucial nutrition and diet are to general health, neural health and mental health. By presenting a succinct book that combines all of the central medical concepts of nutrition with psychological strategies for maintaining a host of new dietary, wellness, health, weight management and lifestyle choices & behaviors, Dr. Wright has found a unique, logical, and flexible method of answering the three most crucial questions when it comes to diet, nutrition, health, wellness, weight and mental health: (1) "what should I eat" (2) "how should I eat it" (3) "why should I eat it"; in a single book!

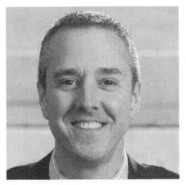

Christopher M. Palmer, MD, Board Certified Psychiatrist, Harvard Psychiatric Expert on The Ketogenic Diet

This lifestyle, health, wellness, weight loss, nutrition & diet book could not be conceived and written at a more prescient time than during a pandemic that stresses even the most hearty and stable among us. It is well known in the field of mental health that what we ingest has a direct and observable effect on our psychological wellbeing and functioning. The building blocks of all essential neurotransmitters are vitamins, minerals and amino acids that are found in sensible and healthy meal plans; but often we, as individuals, and as a society, make accomplishing this more complicated than it needs to be. Dr. Wright's book herein brilliantly breaks down the roadmap to success in both being and eating healthy to a few simple and easily achievable steps attainable in a reasonable time frame. The Nutrient Diet is a must read for anyone who wishes to take a more holistic approach to better living and improved satisfaction with their daily lives and mental functioning.

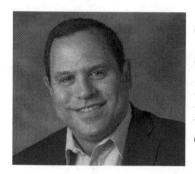 Todd M. Antin, MD, Board Certified in Adult, Addiction, Forensic & Geriatric Psychiatry, Emory Quadruple Board Certified Expert in Psychiatry

For those who wish to maintain or improve their health by eating properly, Dr. Wright's book *The Nutrient Diet*, informative and inspirational from a medical clinician's perspective, is an excellent place to start. From a biblical perspective, Genesis 9:3 says, "Everything that lives and moves will be food for you. Just as I gave you the green plants, I now give you everything." This statement is self-explanatory. However, additional warnings are found in Proverbs 23:20–21. These verses warn us not to be gluttonous in our consumption of food or drink. Dr. Wright splendidly reminds us that we are what we eat and that all dietary consumption should be done in moderation. In just twelve short weeks, by following Dr.

Wright's instructions, starting with a balanced consumption of water and ending with bonus general health and mental health nuggets, you will be able to bring your life to a state of both physical and mental health excellence. I thank God for blessing us with someone (who happens to be my son) who wrote such an enlightening book.

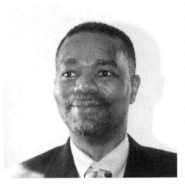

Pastor Harlis R. Wright, Master of Science, Biology; Master of Divinity, Columbia Theological Seminary Pastor, Faith Presbyterian Church (Pine Bluff, Arkansas) Science professor, thirty-five years

About Dr. David

Dr. David A. Wright achieved his MD in July of 2010, graduating Suma Cum Laude [4.0 GPA] from Xavier University School of Medicine. His primary emphases in medical school were forensic psychiatry, addiction psychiatry (addiction medicine), and neurology. While attending medical school, Dr. Wright concurrently completed 3 Masters degrees back to back: an MHSA in healthcare law and policy, an MBA in healthcare administration and an MM in healthcare management. After completing his MD and three Masters degrees,

Dr. Wright became a Forensic Psychiatric Consultant for the largest psychiatric practice in the southeastern United States, PACT Atlanta (since 2010). Instead of pursing a residency in psychiatry Dr. Wright chose to study and train in disciplines that were more in line with the techniques used by the Father and Uncle of Psychiatry, Dr. Sigmund Freud (The Father of Psychiatry) and Dr. Milton Erickson (The Uncle of Psychiatry), respectively. As such, he chose to approach mental health from a more natural, holistic, root cause-based, logic-centered and analytical outlook instead of choosing an approach primarily based on handing out pills to simply address the surface symptoms rather than addressing the underlying, root causes (which is how psychiatry is generally practiced today). Dr. Wright believes that society needs more real solutions, not more pills. Finally, in 2016, Dr. Wright completed his formal training in those disciplines and opened his first practice, MLC Of Greater Atlanta, in Decatur, Georgia, across the street from Emory DeKalb Medical Center. Dr. Wright opened his 2nd practice, Atlanta Coaching & Hypnotherapy Associates (Also Known as Atlanta Coaching), in 2018.

Website Info: www.mlcoga.com
　　　　　　www.atlantacoaching.com

Dr. David A. Wright is the clinical director of MLC of Greater Atlanta [MLCOGA] and Atlanta Coaching & Hypnotherapy Associates [ACHA]. MLC of Greater Atlanta specializes in helping clients who have been diagnosed with the following disorders and conditions, among others: anxiety disorders, adjustment disorders, grief, stress disorders, obsessive compulsive disorder, sleep disorders, panic disorders, phobias, mood disorders, mild to moderate depression, ADD/ADHD, PTSD, personality disorders, learning disabilities, and childhood and adolescent behavioral issues without the use of medications or psychiatric pharmaceutical agents. MLC of Greater Atlanta specializes in helping clients who desire to lose weight, quit smoking, drop destructive habits, change life direction, improve relationships, achieve success and make permanent, long-lasting positive life changes. Atlanta Coaching & Hypnotherapy Associates is primarily focused on providing hypnosis and hypnotherapy.

Dr. Wright is a Physician (i.e., an M.D.), a Board Certified Hypnotherapist, a Board Certified NLP Practitioner, a Board Certified Coach, & a Board Certified Time Line Therapy ® Practitioner who specializes in Non-Pharmacologic, root cause-based, logic-centered, psychoanalytic methods of helping individuals and groups to achieve positive changes and breakthroughs. Dr. Wright is presently accepting new clients and referrals. Dr. Wright also provides consulting services to other healthcare professionals and is a featured speaker and corporate trainer. He is an expert in the areas of "Change Management", "Personal & Professional Development" and "Performance Improvement."

Dr. Wright's current and upcoming books include (1) Sweet Potato Pie for the Spirit, Soul & Psyche (a self-improvement & self-empowerment book) (2) Tomato Bisque for the Brain (a self-improvement & self-empowerment book) (3) The Nutrient Diet (a diet, nutrition, health, wellness, weight loss, weight management and lifestyle management book based on "Cognitive Behavioral" approaches and the psychology of habit formation) (4) The Universal Secrets (a self-improvement & self-empowerment book) (5) Alternative, Holistic & Psychoanalytic Mental Health Approaches (a book for those seeking therapies and life solutions without the use of psychotropic medications). Dr. Wright also has additonal books in progress on a variety of subjects and topics.

CONTENTS

FOREWORD

Dr. Wright's new lifestyle, health, wellness, nutrition, and diet book, *The Nutrient Diet*, could not have come at a better time in history. Nutrition and diet are the building blocks of all metabolic activity, and they form the underpinnings of both general and mental health. I have been using ketogenic diets to treat patients with psychiatric disorders, ranging from major depressive disorder, to bipolar disorder, to schizophrenia, for almost two decades. Because of this, I understand all too well just how crucial nutrition and diet are to general health, neural health, and mental health.

By presenting a succinct book that combines all the central medical concepts of nutrition with psychological strategies for maintaining a host of new dietary, wellness, health, and lifestyle choices and behaviors, Dr. Wright has found a unique, logical, and flexible method of answering the two most crucial questions when it comes to diet, nutrition, health, wellness, medicine, and mental health—"What should I eat?" and "How should I eat?"—in a single book.

The Nutrient Diet will make creating new health and wellness habits practical and easy while providing creative psychology-based methods of maintaining these lifestyle-based behaviors after they have been developed. I highly recommend this thoughtful and carefully crafted book to anyone with a desire to make more well-informed lifestyle-based choices on a consistent basis—regardless of individual health or mental health status. Furthermore, I appreciate the fact that Dr. Wright has included many of the key research studies, clinical trials, and academic articles that help to form the basis of the ketogenic diet.

A fully balanced diet and nutritional approach is vital to the maintenance of good health, and an organized, logical, sensible approach to lifestyle choices, with an emphasis on the psychology of behavior, is a requirement when employing a ketogenic approach.

Christopher M. Palmer, MD, Board-Certified Psychiatrist

Assistant Professor of Psychiatry at Harvard Medical School

Directory of Postgraduate and Continuing Education, McLean Hospital

Research Physician, Behavioral Psychopharmacology Research Laboratory

Research Physician, the Sleep Research Laboratory

Leadership, advisory, and strategic planning committees of Harvard Medical School

Leadership, advisory, and strategic planning committees, Partners Healthcare

Leadership, advisory, and strategic planning committees, the Massachusetts Medical Society

Leadership, advisory, and strategic planning committees, ACCME

CEO and Medical Director

Columnist, "Advancing Psychiatry," *Psychology Today*

Editor, *Journal of Clinical Psychiatry*

Editor, *Journal of Addiction Research and Therapy*

Editor, *Journal of Physiological Anthropology*

Editor, *International Journal of Depression and Anxiety*

Editor, *Journal of Diabetes and Clinical Research*

Editor, *Nutritional Neuroscience*

Psychiatric expert on the ketogenic diet

Author of the following book chapters:

C. M. Palmer and H. G. Pope H.G. Jr., "Antiepileptic Drugs," *The New Oxford Textbook of Psychiatry*, eds. M. G. Gelder, J. J. Lopez-Ibor Jr., and N. Andreason (New York: Oxford University Press, 2000): 1326–33.

C. M. Palmer and M. B. Leslie, "Adult Mental Health," in *Lesbian, Gay, Bisexual, and Transgender Healthcare: A Clinical Guide to Preventive, Primary, and Specialist Care*, eds. K. L. Eckstrand and J. M. Ehrenfeld (Springer Switzerland, 2016), 201–32.

A. Cruz, J. Torrence, and C. Palmer, "Shame in Secrecy in the Psychiatric Encounter," in *Sociocultural Psychiatry: A Casebook and Curriculum*, eds. N. Trin and J. Chen (Oxford: Oxford University Press, forthcoming).

Awards and Academic Citations

Phi Beta Kappa (awarded during junior year), Phi Beta Kappa Society, Academic Achievement, 1990

Community Academic Recognition Award, Lafayette Chamber of Commerce, Academic Achievement and Community Service, 1991

Phi Kappa Phi, the Honor Society of Phi Kappa Phi, Academic Achievement, 1991

Dr. Richard S. Brookings Medical School Prize, Washington University, Academic Achievement, 1993

Honors Graduate Award, Missouri State Medical Association, Academic Achievement, 1995

APA/Glaxo Wellcome Fellowship, American Psychiatric Association, Leadership, 1997–98

AMA Foundation Leadership Award, American Medical Association, 2003

FOREWORD

This lifestyle, health, wellness, nutrition, and diet book could not be conceived and written at a more prescient time than during a pandemic that stresses even the most hearty and stable among us.

It is well-known in the field of mental health that what we ingest has a direct and observable effect on our psychological well-being and functioning.

The building blocks of all essential neurotransmitters are vitamins, minerals, and amino acids, which are found in foods that are part of a sensible and healthy meal plan, but often we, both as individuals and as a society, make it more complicated than it needs to be to include these nutrients in our diets.

Dr. Wright's book brilliantly offers a road map to success in both being healthy and eating healthy to a few simple and easily achievable steps attainable within a reasonable time frame.

The Nutrient Diet is a must-read for anyone who wishes to take a more holistic approach to better living and who wishes to have improved satisfaction with their daily lives and their mental functioning.

Todd M. Antin, MD, Board Certified in Adult, Addiction, Forensic, and Geriatric Psychiatry

Chief Medical Officer, PACT Atlanta

Medical Director, Department of Psychiatry, Emory Decatur Hospital

Adjunct Clinical Assistant Professor, Department of Psychiatry and Behavioral Sciences, Morehouse School of Medicine

Faculty Member, Emory Health Network, Emory University

Clinical Instructor in the Department of Psychiatry, Philadelphia College of Osteopathic Medicine

Adjunct Clinical Assistant Professor in the Department of Physician Assistant Studies, Mercer University College of Pharmacy and Health Sciences

Behavioral Health Medical Director, Department of Psychiatry, Emory Decatur Hospital

Designated one of the United States' Top Psychiatrists by the Consumers' Research Council of America, 2012–19

Elected to Distinguished Fellow Status in the American Psychiatric Association, December 2003

Named one of Atlanta's Top Doctors by *Atlanta Magazine*, 1999–2019 (in all printed issues)

Recognized in *America's Top Doctors*, a national publication of Castle Connolly, 2000–17

Graduate Medical Education Committee Member, Emory Decatur

Physician Health and Wellness Committee Member, Emory Decatur

Executive Leadership Committee Member, Emory Decatur

Clinical trial investigator for dozens of psychiatric drugs and psychiatric disorders, including Prozac (Lilly), CP-118,954 (Pfizer), sertindole (Abbott), venlafaxine (Wyeth-Ayerst), adatanserin (Wyeth-Ayerst), Ziprasidone (Pfizer), Serzone (Bristol Myers Squibb), metrifonate (Miles), flesinoxan (Solvay), Revia (DuPont Merck), Celexa (Forest), Aripiprazole (Otsuka), Risperdal (Janssen), Reminyl (Janssen), Lexapro (Forest), memantine (Forest), MK-073

(Merck), Depakote/Zyprexa (Eli Lilly), Lamictal (GlaxoSmithKline [GSK]), aripiprazole (Bristol Myers Squibb), Seroquel (Astra Zeneca), paliperidone ER (Janssen), Xanax XR (Pfizer), VNS (Cyberonics), paliperidone palmitate (clinical protocol R092670-SCH-4003), psychiatry genotypes (Amplichip), Vivitrol (Alkermes Victory Study), Nuedexta (Prism Avanir Study), Pharmacogenomic Allele study (DART [Diagnosing Adverse Drug Reactions Registry]), Valbenazine/Tardive Dyskinesia (Neurocrine RE-KINECT Study EVA-19350), pimavanserin (Acadia ACP-103-034), dTMS (Brainsway), Marinus (Otsuka), Abilify Mycite (Otsuka), cariprazine (Allergan), and TRD (treatment-resistant depression) (Axsome).

FOREWORD

For those who wish to maintain or improve their health by eating properly, Dr. Wright's book *The Nutrient Diet*, informative and inspirational from a medical clinician's perspective, is an excellent place to start.

From a biblical perspective, Genesis 9:3 says, "Everything that lives and moves will be food for you. Just as I gave you the green plants, I now give you everything." This statement is self-explanatory. However, additional warnings are found in Proverbs 23:20–21. These verses warn us not to be gluttonous in our consumption of food or drink.

Dr. Wright splendidly reminds us that we are what we eat and that all dietary consumption should be done in moderation. In just twelve short weeks, by following Dr. Wright's instructions, starting with a balanced consumption of water and ending with bonus general health and mental health nuggets, you will be able to bring your life to a state of both physical and mental health excellence.

I thank God for blessing us with someone (who happens to be my son) who wrote such an enlightening book.

Pastor Harlis R. Wright, Master of Science, Biology; Master of Divinity, Columbia Theological Seminary

Pastor, Faith Presbyterian Church (Pine Bluff, Arkansas)

Science professor, thirty-five years

INTRODUCTION

The idea for *The Nutrient Diet* came from my noticing so many people jumping from diet to diet, year to year, decade after decade, and seeing them essentially stay at the same weight (and, in many cases, grow even larger). Since the 1980s, I've observed literally hundreds of diet plans come and go. Although a few of them, such as Weight Watchers, Jenny Craig, and Nutrisystem, have appeared to stand the test of time, most of them seem to come and go like the wind. The more popular ones are all the rage for about two years, and then they quickly vanish into the obscurity of the diet book section of Barnes & Noble, or else they enter the lonely confines of the bargain book rack at Books-A-Million. As these once-praised diet books fade into obscurity, so do the hopes and dreams of every person attempting to lose weight, control their appetite, manage his or her waistline, make healthier choices, or create a new lifestyle. I've gotten to see this up close and personal within my own family, within myself, and within the clients of my practices.

Through all these observations, and by taking an analytic approach to them both singularly and in aggregate, I came to the conclusion that the vast majority of these diets fail because they expect the individual to make too many primary changes at once. In essence, they expect the person to change overnight—which rarely happens anywhere in nature (including within humanity). It is true that plans, goals, and objectives tend to fail when they require too many steps too quickly. I base this opinion on the simplicity principle: the simpler something is to set up and begin, the more likely one is to consistently continue (i.e., perpetuate) it. The reverse of this is the complexity principle: the more complicated something is to set up, begin, and perpetuate, the more likely one is to abruptly discontinue (i.e., abandon) it.

Here's an example. Let's say you ask your five-year-old to begin brushing her teeth herself each morning. If the steps involved in that process include four simple actions (i.e., rinsing the toothbrush, adding the toothpaste, brushing the teeth adequately, and rinsing the toothbrush once again), which together take about two minutes, then the child is likely to be able to easily learn them and then repeat them every morning—right?—just like most children learn to do for themselves. But let's consider a different scenario. What if the following steps were involved in brushing your teeth each morning: (1) Rinsing the toothbrush for about five minutes, using a solution that you have to create each morning using salt, water, peroxide, and bleach. (2) Creating homemade toothpaste each morning out of fresh mint, baking soda, gel, and an essential oil, which takes about five minutes. (3) Brushing every single tooth for about fifteen seconds on each side, knowing that each tooth has two sides. (4) Rinsing your mouth out with water seven times, taking about five minutes. (5) Rinsing the toothbrush once again for about five minutes, using a solution that you have to create each morning using salt, water, peroxide, and bleach. Altogether, this combination of five steps would take the following amount of time:

- Step 1—toothbrush rinsing, five minutes
- Step 2—creating homemade toothpaste, five minutes
- Step 3—brushing every single tooth for thirty seconds each; with twenty teeth, this equates to ten minutes
- Step 4—mouth rinsing, five minutes
- Step 5—second round of toothbrush rinsing, five minutes

That's a grand total of thirty minutes to brush your teeth every morning, and then another thirty minutes to clean them at night before bed. Honestly, if brushing one's teeth were that tedious and complicated, do you think that the average four- or five-year-old would pick up the habit?

Do you ever wonder why many people didn't regularly and consistently brush their teeth before toothbrushes, hot running water, and toothpaste were affordable and widely available? You've got it! Because it was so tedious (i.e., challenging) to install the habit as a new behavior. The easier something is to repeat consistently enough to become a habit, routine, and/or ritual, the more likely it is to become part of the style of your daily life and, hence, your lifestyle. Therefore, in order for something to become a part of your lifestyle, it *must* be fairly easy to complete, easily reproducible consistently, and constantly rewarding (in this case, the rewards include white teeth, good breath, and an attractive, approachable smile). A similar analogy would be of bowling balls rolling down a lane at a local bowling alley. Which ball is more likely to make it to the end, one that is a complete simple sphere (i.e., perfectly round/circular) or one with ornate designs and projections coming from it? Of course, the simple circular sphere always wins the race. In fact, the other "ball" will probably fail even to roll at all, right? There's a *reason* why bowling balls are perfectly round, right? So that there is little to no friction to decrease the velocity as they travel down the bowling lane (i.e., accomplish their purpose).

The same is true of most diets (i.e., lifestyle modification plans [LMPs]). Because diets are generally complex, even when someone strives to make them easy, they are difficult to permanently install as a habit, routine, and/or ritual. Just think about it! The average diet plan requires the following steps, at a minimum: (1) You have to notice a book, commercial, or other advertisement. (2) You have to be engaged by it enough to lend it your attention. (3) You have to take the time to respond to the book, commercial, or other advertisement. (4) You have listen to the sales pitch. (5) You have to decide that the diet is doable and worth the costs. (6) You have to decide that you *are* going to do it (i.e., set a diet date). (7) You have to agree and then purchase the diet program.

All that, and you haven't even started the diet yet! Then, you have to *start* the diet after the supplies have arrived, you've checked in at the diet center, or you've bought the foods that you need to follow the diet on your own. That's why it's so difficult for the vast majority of individuals to start, continue, and complete a diet or other lifestyle plan.

So, what's the solution? Well, for one, you need to find something that is doable and able to be perpetuated (i.e., consistently repeated and/or reproducible). Hence, the *chief* characteristic of such a diet has to be *simplicity*.

Think about it like this: What if you were to purchase a new hotel and you, as the owner, had to learn every single service function and job at the hotel (with fifty-four different types of positions at the hotel) just in case an employee called in sick or quit? Would it be easier for you to learn a new job function every week (i.e., learn to do one new job each week) for fifty-four weeks, or would it be easier to learn to do all of them at once (i.e., learn fifty-four different jobs in one week)? Easy answer, right? It would be much easier to learn a new job function each week, and then repeat the ones that you've already learned while learning new ones—until you've mastered all of them over a period of fifty-four weeks.

The same is true for lifestyle changes. You're much more likely to be successful *if* you create and continue *one* new lifestyle choice each week for a certain amount of time. Now all that you have to do is *choose* which lifestyle choices that you'd like to add (or remove) each week for fifty-four weeks! In this case, it's only twelve weeks (i.e., three months). I *always* recommend beginning with the basics, the building blocks. So, start with what you do when you first awaken in the morning, and go from there until you reach the end of the day—until you have the week mapped out. Then you can look at the weekend and go from there to the details that are individualistic in nature. Keep in mind that you *do not* have to make these changes in the order provided here, although I would suggest this order as it makes things easier.

Each chapter that follows represents a weekly change in life(style)—one change per week. You could begin either at the beginning of the year (i.e., in January) or at any other time. There's plenty of room for *flexibility*.

The Nutrient Diet is a completely new, bold, different psychological approach to diet, health, wellness, and weight-management habits. It's a lifestyle book for general and mental health based on sound psychological principles. *The Nutrient Diet* is 50 percent about diet and nutrition and 50 percent about cognitive and behavioral psychological strategies for eating behaviors, dieting, impulse control, and habit formation. It's the first book of its kind to take a cognitive behavioral (i.e., psychological) approach to diet, nutrition, health, wellness, and lifestyle management. It truly is a trendsetter in the diet, health, wellness, medicine, nutrition, and lifestyle fields. Not only does *The Nutrient Diet* show and explain what you need to eat, but it also explains *how* you should eat it—based on sound, tested scientific data and psychological principles. And it does this in a way that allows you to make lifestyle changes easily, naturally, and progressively so that you don't get overwhelmed.

I've used these principles, techniques, and methods of habit formation to help my clients who are seeking abundance, empowerment, courage, confidence, prosperity, and direction to successfully change careers, double their incomes, move past procrastination and stagnation, lose substantial amounts of weight, and re-create happiness and joy in their lives. *The Nutrient Diet* shows you how to use your thoughts, feelings, moods, actions, reactions, habits, and belief systems so that they become allies in your weight-management, diet, and lifestyle goals. Together, these tools, methods, resources, strategies, and approaches will positively change the trajectory of your life—while simultaneously adding joy, happiness, and fulfillment to it! The keys to diet, weight management, and impulse control are habit and ritual creation, formation, and sustainment. *The Nutrient Diet* will help you build a daily self-care regimen that works for you. It will help you to care for your mind and body in a way that empowers you daily, while preventing frustration, stagnation, and exhaustion. And, if you use it with my other books (which have tools to help support a mindset that encompasses healthy habits, choices, and rituals), which introduce and draw upon alternative mental health and wellness techniques such as hypnosis, hypnotherapy, mindfulness, mind-setting, NLP (neurolinguistic programming), and Time Line Therapy®, then you will have a foolproof tool for a healthier, happier lifestyle and greater well-being.

Your dietary and wellness history definitely has helped to shape who and what you are today. But the negative aspects of your history don't have to define who you are in the future. You, and you alone, get to define, develop, and defend your desires and your destiny! And you've started the journey to determine, develop, and define your desires and your destiny by using the techniques, methods, and resources that are introduced here!

Along the way, you might slip. You might even fall. But if you continue to employ the techniques and methods that you've learned here, you will never, ever stay on the ground! You'll become *tougher*! You'll become *stronger*! You'll become a *fighter*! And, that's what it takes to win the battle for your *destiny*! It truly is all about those little steps that you take on a daily basis. I like to call them habits.

CHAPTER 1

Water

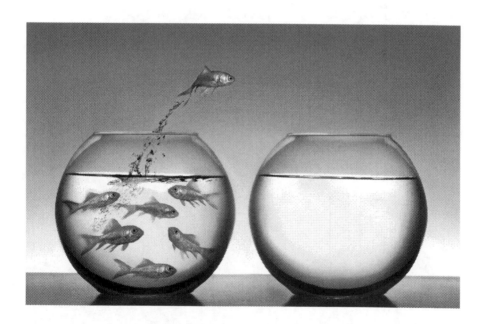

Why start with water? Well over 50 percent of your body is water. In fact, almost two-thirds (i.e., 66 percent) of your body is composed of water. How is that? Well, the basic building block of all life is the cell, and cells are filled with a water-like fluid called the cytoplasm or fluid of the cell. These cells are arranged into cooperative groups and/or sheets called tissues, which contain additional fluids. And these tissues (i.e., sheets of similar cells) are arranged into even more specialized groups to form organs, which tend to hold and circulate even more liquids/fluids. These organs are contained within sacs of fluids, and they communicate with one another through chemicals that travel through tubes (blood vessels, etc.) that are filled with other specialized fluids, namely, blood and plasma.

So, the general layout of the human body is the following:

(1) Cell
(2) Fluid
(3) Cell
(4) Fluid
(5) Cell
(6) Fluid

The cells are bathed in, are affected by, and contain fluids! Everything happens by, within, and through the use of a *fluid*. After all, according to evolution, all cellular life began in a fluid—the ocean.

Since water (i.e., a fluid), in addition to the cell, is the *basis of living*, we have to start there. Not only does water make metabolism possible in your body, but it also helps to eliminate the stuff that your body doesn't need, both through osmosis and other, more energetic and specific processes. Hence, you need an adequate exchange of water to get rid of the things that you don't want to hold in your body, such as toxins, waste products of metabolism, sugars, carbohydrates, and fats. You have to constantly and consistently filter water throughout the body (using your tissues, such as your kidneys) in order to get rid of these things. And the only way to do this is to continuously bring in water and continuously remove it so that your body always has new, fresh water.

It might be helpful to think of your body as a fishbowl, a fish tank, or an aquarium. How would your body work and function if it looked like a fishbowl in which the water hadn't been changed for a year? It probably wouldn't be an environment amenable to the healthy living of fish after a few weeks, right? This is to say nothing of a few months. That's why fish tanks and aquariums (where the water is constantly being filtered) were created. If you don't consume a consistent amount of fresh water, then your body will be like a fish tank with water that's been sitting around for years. It's *not* a healthy environment for cells, tissues, and organs to live in, communicate, thrive in, and survive. Just look at the following pictures to get a sense of the differences.

Which of these environments would you prefer to live in? Which ones look the healthiest to you? Which environments do you think would be the best for fending off harmful bacteria, viruses, and disease? Clearly, the cleaner ones would be environments where life is more likely to thrive and be sustained for longer periods. So, we have to begin with water.

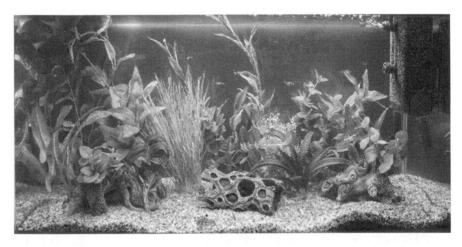

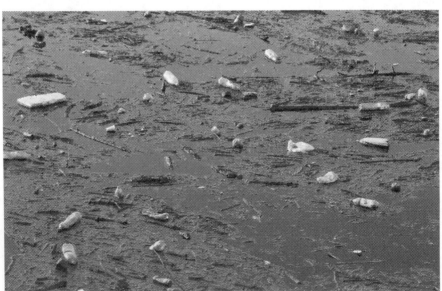

What type of water are we talking about, and how much do we need? According to Healthline, "Health authorities commonly recommend eight 8-ounce glasses, which equals about 2 liters, or half a gallon. This is called the 8×8 rule and is very easy to remember." However, many health professionals suggest that you should sip on water throughout the day. And many researchers in recent years have suggested that you don't actually need to consume eight glasses of water per day. The amount of water that you consume each day should be based on your height and weight (i.e., your size and/or BMI). But if you are an average-sized adult who has an average amount of daily bodily activity, then about four to six glasses (i.e., eight to twelve cups) of water each day should be sufficient. You should adjust this amount as you move to the right or the left of these averages. For instance, if you're a thirty-five-year-old male who stands at 6'3" and weighs 220 pounds, and if you work out one to two hours each day, then you should probably consume close to eight glasses of water per day. But if you're a fifty-five-year-old female who is 5'4" and 135 pounds, and if you have a fairly sedentary lifestyle (and a low daily caloric intake), then you'd probably be better off consuming about four glasses of water per day. Does that make sense? In other words, not everyone should necessarily be using a one-size-fits-all system for daily water consumption. In addition, your daily water consumption should also take into account your health status (BMI), any chronic conditions that you have (hypertension, diabetes, renal failure, etc.), your daily caloric intake, your daily caloric expenditure (amount of exercise and/or physical activity), and any prescription medications and/or supplements that you are currently taking. So, if you take a blood-pressure-lowering agent for hypertension (such as hydrochlorothiazide, Lisinopril, or amlodipine), then you might need to be at the higher end of the water consumption spectrum. If in doubt, then consult your licensed healthcare provider.

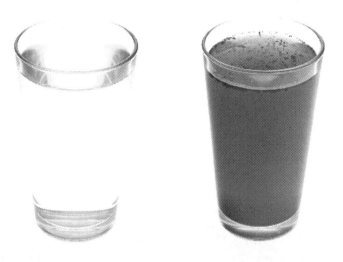

How does water help you lose weight? The following is according to Healthline:

According to two studies, drinking 17 ounces (500 ml) of water can temporarily boost metabolism by 24–30%.[1]

The researchers estimated that drinking 68 ounces (2 liters) in one day increased energy expenditure by about 96 calories per day. Additionally, it may be beneficial to drink cold water because your body will need to expend more calories to heat the water to body temperature. Drinking water about a half hour before meals can also reduce the number of calories you end up consuming, especially in

---

[1]   Boschmann M, Steiniger J, Hille U, et al. Water-induced thermogenesis. J Clin Endocrinol Metab. 2003;88(12):6015-6019. doi:10.1210/jc.2003-030780. Retrieved from https://www.ncbi.nlm.nih.gov/pubmed/14671205

Davy BM, Dennis EA, Dengo AL, Wilson KL, Davy KP. Water consumption reduces energy intake at a breakfast meal in obese older adults. J Am Diet Assoc. 2008;108(7):1236-1239. doi:10.1016/j.jada.2008.04.013. Retrieved from https://www.ncbi.nlm.nih.gov/pubmed/18589036

Van Walleghen EL, Orr JS, Gentile CL, Davy BM. Pre-meal water consumption reduces meal energy intake in older but not younger subjects. Obesity (Silver Spring). 2007;15(1):93-99. doi:10.1038/oby.2007.506. Retrieved from https://www.ncbi.nlm.nih.gov/pubmed/17228036

Van Walleghen EL, Orr JS, Gentile CL, Davy BM. Pre-meal water consumption reduces meal energy intake in older but not younger subjects. Obesity (Silver Spring). 2007;15(1):93-99. doi:10.1038/oby.2007.506. Retrieved from https://www.ncbi.nlm.nih.gov/pubmed/17228036

Bjarnadottir, MS, RDN. How Drinking More Water Can Help You Lose Weight. Healthline, 2017. Retrieved from https://www.healthline.com/nutrition/drinking-water-helps-with-weight-loss

older individuals. One study showed that dieters who drank 17 ounces (500 ml) of water before each meal lost 44% more weight over 12 weeks, compared to those who didn't. Overall, it seems that drinking adequate amounts of water, particularly before meals, may have a significant weight loss benefit, especially when combined with a healthy diet.[2]

Basically, water allows your body to stave off appetite and to complete metabolic functions, thereby burning calories, while allowing your body the fluid volume needed to expel wastes and toxins and perform other regulatory functions. In addition, according to Healthline, increased water intake also helps to prevent constipation, cancer, and kidney stones.

Some sources use the following chart as a general guide to daily water consumption:

---

[2] Kris Gunnars, "How Much Water Should You Drink Per Day?" Healthline, last updated November 5, 2020, https://www.healthline.com/nutrition/how-much-water-should-you-drink-per-day.

[3] Ashley Marcin, "How Much Water You Need to Drink," Healthline, last updated March 7, 2019, https://www.healthline.com/health/how-much-water-should-I-drink.

Demographic	Daily recommended amount of water (from drinks)
▪ children 4–8 years old	5 cups, or 40 total ounces
▪ children 9–13 years old	7–8 cups, or 56–64 total ounces
▪ children 14–18 years old	8–11 cups, or 64–88 total ounces
▪ men, 19 years and older	13 cups, or 104 total ounces
▪ women, 19 years and older	9 cups, or 72 total ounces
▪ pregnant women	10 cups, or 80 total ounces
▪ breastfeeding women	13 cups, or 104 total ounces[2]

Also, keep in mind that about two cups of water makes up a glass of water. If you consume water by the glass, then just take the number of cups and divide it by 2 (and vice versa). Most adults don't consume water by the cup—they generally consume water by the bottle, by the glass, or by the gallon.

By the way, insufficient water consumption can lead to dehydration (and hypernatremia), a low-energy state. Dehydration can lead to any of the following health conditions and/or disease states:

- confusion
- mood changes
- depression
- anxiety
- overeating
- constipation
- kidney stones
- shock
- death.

However, drinking too much water can lead to hyponatremia (i.e., low sodium/salt), which can lead to any of the following health conditions and/or disease states:

- confusion
- headache
- fatigue
- nausea or vomiting
- irritability
- muscle spasms, cramps, or weakness
- seizures
- coma
- psychosis
- death.[4]

---

[4]   Ibid.

So, the goal here is water *balance*, not just water consumption (which is what has typically been championed in the past). And there's a huge difference between the two concepts in terms of lifestyle choices.

Certain foods do tend to contain a higher water content. They include the following:

- melons
- spinach
- cucumbers
- green peppers
- berries
- cauliflower
- radishes
- celery.[5]

Furthermore, water allows your body to move nutrients, break down compounds, and move reactions forward that allow your body to use the vitamins and minerals that are present in the foods and drinks you consume. This is especially true for the water-soluble vitamins, such as the B vitamins (B_1, B_2, B_3, B_4, B_5, B_6, B_{12}, etc.) and vitamin C, and the minerals.

Finally, the type of water that you consume is extremely important. This is why I would not recommend that you consume tap water! One more time: Do *not* drink

---

[5]   Ibid.

tap water! There are many reasons why you should not drink tap water. However, the most important reason is that you have no idea what's in it. Many people might argue that you might not know what's in a bottle of water you purchase. There is truth to that statement. Therefore, the best method is to have a water filtration system that you have researched and can trust. Outside of that, you need to find a source for water that you trust. At the end of the day, we don't really know what is in *anything* 100 percent.

The most common water filtration systems use one or more of the following methods to clean (i.e., purify) the water:

- activated carbon filters
- ion exchange units
- reverse osmosis units
- distillation units.[6]

However, it should be noted that no one water filtration system will eliminate all contaminants. And most water filtration systems need to be cleaned, maintained, and serviced regularly in order to maintain the level of water purification as advertised. In my opinion, a hybrid filtration system is probably best. In addition, many

---

[6]   Sabrina Felson, "Drinking Water Quality: What You Need to Know," WebMD, accessed October 23, 2018, https://www.webmd.com/women/safe-drinking-water.

people are now choosing to consume only alkalinized water. However, the jury is still out on the benefits of drinking alkalinized (i.e., alkaline) water. While acidic water can damage bodily structures, basic water (i.e., alkaline water) can cause deposits to form in bodily structures. So, you have to have a pH balance. Pure water has a pH of 7.0, which is optimal, but tap water often fails to reach a pH of 7.0 and may have a pH as low as 4.0, which is on the acidic side. For these reasons, I recommend either the consumption of water from a tested, trustable water filtration system or the consumption of bottled water from a trusted source. Additionally, acidic and basic (i.e., alkaline) substances have the power to kill harmful organisms—which is how your saliva and stomach acid help to prevent disease. For instance, if you use your diet to make your body fluids less acidic, it could backfire and neutralize your body's ability to fight off harmful organisms and/or infectious diseases. Therefore, I would recommend the consumption of water as close to a pH of 7.0 as possible, from a trusted source.

So, for week 1, start changing your water consumption habits. Honestly, if you learn but a single thing from *The Nutrient Diet, do learn to change, monitor and control your water consumption and water balance habits.* Your water balance ritual is the single most important modifiable factor for your health, weight, and longevity.

Take the following water balance steps during week 1: (1) Start your day off with a glass or bottle of water. (2) Have one glass or bottle of water in between other beverages. (3) Have one-half to one glass or bottle of water an hour before each meal in order to pad your appetite, which will lead you to consume less food. (4) Drink water with snacks. (5) Dilute other beverages with ice and water. (6) Finish the day off with a glass of water.

And remember, although many experts suggest drinking water at room temperature (or even water that is slightly warm), your body actually burns a greater number of calories when you drink colder water—because it has to expend calories (by increasing the number of chemical reactions) in order to maintain your body temperature while you are actively lowering it by consuming something that is cold. Remember: Your body burns calories (and, hence, fat) in order to produce energy and maintain temperature. That's why babies have such a high percentage of body weight as fat and, more specifically, as brown fat.

The mission for week 1 is simple: Change your water consumption and balance habits! Don't worry about any other habits during week 1! The only goal is to change your water rituals! We'll tackle food, soft drinks, number of meals per day, snack habits, exercise, and other lifestyle habits in later chapters, one week at a time.

CHAPTER 2

Sugars & Sweeteners

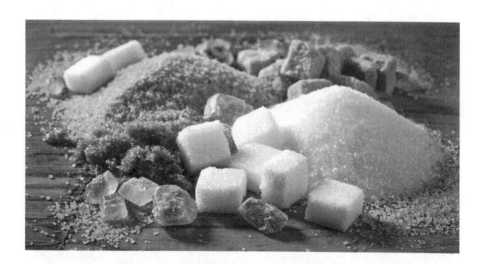

The next most important thing to do with regard to your diet is to focus on is *sugar*. Two of the most important sets of substances in your body are proteins and sugars. Why do I say this? Three key reasons: (1) communication, (2) security, and (3) energy. Just as our culture needs energy (i.e., power), communication tools (i.e., computers, phones, and televisions), and security (i.e., physical armies and military personnel, antivirus software, home alarm systems, and security pass codes and PINs), so do our cells, tissues, organs, and bodies. None of it is by accident. It's all by careful design and according to an intricate plan arising from time-tested strategies. Just as we use language, sounds, symbols, and expressions to communicate meaning, our cells and tissues use sugars (and proteins and, hence, enzymes) to do the same thing. And they use them between one another to trade energy and signals.

The backbone of organic life and, hence, of organic chemistry is carbon. Organic life-forms use molecules composed of carbon in order to communicate and trade. Flowers and plants take in carbon dioxide and sunlight from the environment and give off proteins, sugars, and oxygen. Then, animals take in these proteins, sugars, and oxygen and give off metabolic waste products and carbon dioxide. These metabolic waste products and carbon dioxide are then retaken up by the environment (by plants) so they can be recycled. In addition, animals are also able to recycle some substances such as sugars, carbohydrates, proteins (and, hence, enzymes), and neurotransmitters (such as acetyl choline, dopamine, serotonin, and epinephrine).

The basic concept is that cycles of metabolic activity are formed between the sun, the gases of the earth, and the earth's plants and animals. Sugars are by-products of these cycles, and they help facilitate the energy and signal exchanges needed to fulfill the cycles. However, transferring and trading energy and messages requires energy. So, all energy and communication transfers are not equal. That's one of the reasons why biochemistry (and, hence, our bodies) uses phosphates, in order to quantify energy production and transfers, in the form of ATP (adenosine triphosphate).

The mammalian body (including the human body) uses sugars for a variety of tasks. Sugars are used for communication between cells (via signals), for energy transfers, and for the building blocks of your body's foundation [which is a combination and organization of cells, tissues, organs, organ systems and fluids]. Sugars are used by cells to communicate using protein channels. Just as channels on a radio or on a TV are used to communicate between the sources of information and the receivers of information, cells and tissues use channels to communicate. And they often use proteins, sugars, and carbohydrates in order to do so.

The important concept here is that your cells need the right sugars to properly communicate with one another expeditiously. If your body has access to simple sugars (and/or proteins), then it can use these as the building blocks for the more complex sugars (and carbohydrates) that are needed by specific cells and tissues. However, if these simpler sugars are not available, then tissues and organs will have to shift their production schedules in order to produce the specific sugars that are needed. They will either have to sequester these from new nutrients that have just been made available (which zaps them from the nutrient pool needed for more immediate processes such as walking, which requires energy) or have to break down more complex molecules (i.e., recycle) in order to reproduce the simpler sugars—which requires additional energy. This is akin to running in circles when nutrient levels are depleted. When this occurs, your tissues and organs may spend more time recycling materials from one form to another than trading the sugars between themselves.

Think of it this way: What if your body's metabolic activities (i.e., communication and complementarity between cells, tissues, and organs) were represented by a relay race on a track, with four runners working together as a team to cover eight hundred meters in a dash, while competing with other teams trying to accomplish the same goal at the same time? The team with the quickest runners and the fastest baton passes will win the race, right? In practice, each team will work together so that each of the four runners runs optimally and also is able to transfer the baton to the next runner with as little loss of time, speed, and momentum as possible, right? Generally speaking, the race elements that represent the greatest opportunities for loss of speed and momentum are the start-off and the pace of each individual runner on the team, along with the time that it takes to pass the baton without losing momentum. Hence, the baton passes are one the greatest opportunities in the relay race to make up time/speed, lose time/speed, and/or maintain time or speed. The same is true within the human body. Moreover, the metabolic "baton passes" that occur within the human body are vitally important to our physiological functioning.

The availability of certain sugars, carbohydrates, and proteins helps to facilitate quick transfers or energy (these are sometimes referred to as rate-limiting factors). Therefore, if and when specific molecules of sugar, carbohydrate, and/or protein are unavailable, then the baton passes (i.e., energy transfers) between cells, tissues, and organs will be delayed until those substances can be produced again. Moreover, having the proper sugars, carbohydrates, and proteins available allows your metabolism, via intricate, interconnected biochemical pathways and cycles, to function smoothly and optimally.

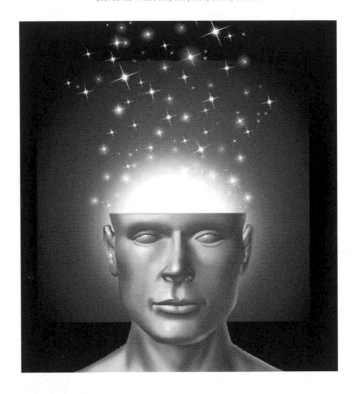

Note that the purer the energy source, the less time your tissues and organs will have to spend on recycling materials and eliminating waste products, and the more time they will have to use for fruitful processes and services. That's why eating *cleanly* is so important. Taking in better, cleaner sugar allows for faster and more-efficient energy transfers and facilitates better communication between cells, tissues, and organs—while also reducing time and energy spent on waste management and elimination. This same concept is illustrated by the octane of the gasoline that you place in your car (if it has a gasoline engine): the higher the octane, the more cleanly the engine burns the fuel.

The third function of sugars is to serve as a building block of your body's foundation. This is where the source and the type of sugars that you intake is perhaps most important. Plants and animals are both dynamic in different ways. Plants are highly dependent upon both the environment (for water and nutrients from the soil) and the sun (for energy). While humans and other animals may not be quite as directly dependent upon the sun (although they are indirectly dependent via plants and other animals that consume plants—and by the need for vitamin D production in order to regulate body calcium levels, etc.), humans are also more dynamic and flexible in terms of nutrients.

Our bodies have the amazing ability to take in energy from a plethora of different sources and use it to perpetuate life. Now, will that life be productive, efficient, and/or meaningful? Well, that's an entirely different discussion. But droughts and famines throughout history have shown that humans can survive for quite some time on very little (e.g., bread and water; tea and crumpets; plants and a water source). Plants can't do that. Try feeding a plant Kool-Aid or fruit juice. Try feeding a flower a neck bone. It just won't work. Plants can't survive on those substances alone. But humans can—at least for a short amount of time.

Our metabolisms use hundreds of metabolic pathways and cycles (which form the basis of the discipline of biochemistry) to transform one substance into another in order to enable the body to use it for some purpose that is beneficial. It's amazing, but it's also a double-edged sword. And that's where we get into trouble.

Let's compare two scenarios. In the first scenario, you have a plant that needs certain nutrients such as sunlight, water, and nitrogen, but all you have available is junk food—Kool-Aid, potato chips, pork rinds, and Twinkies. So, what happens? Well, obviously, the plant dies because, in its simplicity, it doesn't possess the ability to use these sources of energy for its metabolic activities. If a plant doesn't have the most basic of needed energy sources, then it dies. But what about a human?

Well, we have the ability to use almost anything, even junk. So, when fresh water, fresh fish, vitamins and minerals, fresh fruits and vegetables, and other sources of nutrients are unavailable, the human body will do what it can with the "junk" that is available to it. However, the opposite edge of that sword is that what the body creates from that junk will reflect what was available. If you put junk in, then you'll get junk out. While a human may be able to survive for longer than the plant on junk food, his or her health will reflect that he or she fed his or her body junk.

One particular human autoimmune disorder perfectly illustrates this concept, namely, multiple sclerosis (MS)—a relatively new disease in human evolution. In multiple sclerosis, the body's own immune cells attack the material that insulates the nerves. The nerves themselves, which communicate information and energy, are called axons and dendrites. The protective covering (i.e., the insulation for the electrical wires) over the nerves is called the myelin sheath. The myelin sheath protects the axons and dendrites from being damaged by the environment, just like the black covering (i.e., insulation) on wires that lead to appliances protects the flow of electricity from one point to another. But what if the wires to your electronics weren't covered by the insulation around the cord? Well, your electronics would continually encounter damage, and eventually they wouldn't work at all. Our nerves are the same way. If they aren't covered by a myelin sheath (i.e., a protective cord), then they too will undergo constant damage up to the time when the damage is so great that the nerve cells are no longer able to communicate (i.e., transmit signals). That, in turn, leads to loss of nervous function and loss of the ability to sense and, hence, to properly communicate.

Well, what if your nerve cells didn't have the necessary materials to build myelin sheaths around the nerve cells in order to protect the communications between nerves, tissues, and organs? Well, then they would build them out of whatever was available. That is what happens with multiple sclerosis.

The myelin sheath that covers nerves, much like the plastic or rubber cord that covers electrical wires, is principally made up of three substances:

- lipids (i.e., fats/cholesterols), 60 percent to 75 percent
- sugars (i.e., glycolipids/galactocerebrosides)
- proteins (myelin basic protein [MBP]), myelin oligodendrocyte glycoprotein [MOG], proteolipid protein [PLP], and myelin protein zero [MPZ]), 15 percent to 25 percent.

So, what happens if the body doesn't have the pure raw materials to create the myelin sheath that protects nerves and helps to facilitate the required communication between those nerves? As I've already mentioned, because it's the human body, it does what it can with what it has. Therefore, it will attempt to build myelin sheaths out of whatever closest ingredients are available. If it doesn't have the right lipids, sugars, and proteins available, then it will attempt to build the myelin sheath out of whatever it has available—in the same way that a home builder would have to either stop building or use wood or stone instead if he or she were to run out of bricks. And that's just what it does. So, what's the problem then? The problem is evolution.

The same evolutionary forces and processes that have made it unnecessary for plants to use alternative fuel sources (since our planet has previously had plentiful water, nitrogen, sunlight, etc.) have also made our bodies highly specific with regard to the building blocks that it uses to create metabolic structures. For thousands of years, our bodies have essentially used the same types and kinds of nutrients to build and create what they've needed (membranes, tissues, organs, etc.).

Essentially, the same types of lipids, proteins, and sugars have been available to humans for millions of years. However, this hasn't been the case during the last hundred years. During the last hundred years, technology has allowed humanity to create things that we never could have imagined were possible. And those inventions have not eluded the food industry. Today we make foods by combining and creating things that have never been created before, and we consume these things in greater quantities and more often than ever before. If a person from two hundred years ago were to travel to a modern-day grocery store such as Publix or Kroger, such an individual would be utterly lost. Most of us get lost in large grocery stores, and we've been alive for these technological advancements.

Well, let's look at what's available to use these days, as opposed to what was available one hundred or two hundred years ago. Today we have genetically engineered and genetically modified meats and vegetables, along with alternative sugars and sweeteners such as stevia, Truvia, Sweet One, Splenda, xylitol, sorbitol, Sweet 'N Low (saccharin), and Equal (aspartame). It has taken the human body literally millions of years to develop and evolve into what it is today. If your body begins using alternative sources to build what it needs, then what it ends up building could look and function vastly different from what it's been used to for millions of years of our evolution. Herein lies the source of the problem with autoimmune disorders such as multiple sclerosis.

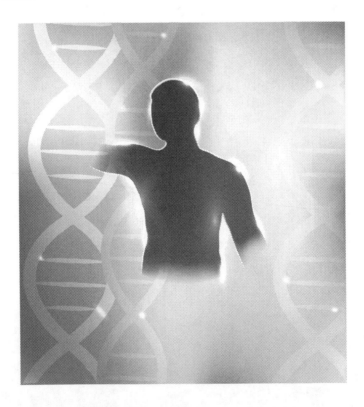

The human body sends thousands upon thousands of protective cells (i.e., immune cells) around the body in order to help fight viruses, prevent bacteria and fungi from taking hold (and fighting them off once they do cause an infection), and destroy cancer cells. The central purpose of many of these immune cells is to notice and eliminate what is foreign to the body, that is, what doesn't belong there. These cells have evolved over millions of years in order to do just that. When your caloric intake consists of substances found naturally within your environment, such as those from nature-grown plants and animals, then your body's cells, tissues, and organs will recognize those substances as part of the normal environment (with the exception of certain infectious organisms, of course) and will help to preserve and protect them. However, if your caloric intake consists of substances not found naturally within your environment (such as genetically engineered and/or modified meats and/or vegetables, strange carbohydrates, and artificial sweeteners and sugar substitutes), then your body's immune cells will detect, attack, and eliminate those substances if they are not being used to produce energy.

So, if a significant majority of your caloric intake consists of genetically engineered meats, strange carbohydrates, and artificial sweeteners and sugar substitutes, then your body's cells, tissues, and organs will do the best they can to break down and/or build up those substances into what they need to create energy and to build bodily structures such as cell membranes, ducts, tissues, and organs. However, there are limits to the body's ability to transform substances, the primary limitation being evolution. Our bodies haven't had enough time to evolve to efficiently and productively use all these artificial, foreign, and novel substances. So, what do our bodies do when these are the only sources of fuel and/or raw materials? They use them. And when our bodies use these building blocks to create tissues, organs, organelles, and cellular structures, our white blood cells can and do identify them as foreign, and attack them. That's the pathogenesis of autoimmune diseases.

In multiple sclerosis, since the person lives off all of these artificial, foreign, and novel substances, the body is forced to use those available substances to build and regenerate membranes, organelles, tissues, and organs. In multiple sclerosis, white blood cells will detect elements within the myelin sheath (be they lipids, sugars, or proteins) as foreign and then attack them. This leads to demyelination (the removal of the myelin sheath by the immune cells) and to neurological dysfunction and disease (i.e., the inability of nervous tissue to properly function and, hence, communicate). This is the reason why you rarely see autoimmune disorders in people (or cultures) with healthier, more natural dietary and lifestyle habits. It's also the reason why you tend to see a higher incidence and prevalence of autoimmune disorders in Westernized cultures, where there is a greater availability of genetically modified and/or engineered foods, strange carbohydrates, and artificial sweeteners and sugar substitutes—that is, artificial, foreign, and novel substances.

If you want to prevent autoimmune disorders, then choose a diet that is as close to human nature (and, hence, our natural environment) as possible—one that consists of more natural foods and fewer processed and/or genetically engineered or genetically modified foods. Sugars are the best place to start.

I would recommend the following in terms of your sugar intake: (1) Intake natural sugars from fruits and plants. (2) Use coconut sugar and organic brown and yellow sugars instead of overly processed sugars. (3) Avoid whitened, bleached, and/or highly processed sugars. (4) Avoid artificial sweeteners such as Sweet 'N Low (contains saccharin), Equal (contains aspartame), Splenda, and Birth Sugar (i.e., xylitol) (the jury is still out on novel sweeteners such as stevia and Truvia). (5) Dilute sugary drinks with filtered water so they are less concentrated. (6) Gradually decrease the concentration of and amount of sugar that you intake daily. (7) If you do intake substances that are high in sugar or contain alternative sweeteners, do so in the morning, when your body is in the process of burning energy as you do work (as opposed to at night/bedtime, when your body is in the process of building things that you will need for tomorrow). (8) Research and explore more-natural alternative sweeteners that don't lead to high glycemic indexes or spikes in blood sugar, such as agave nectar, coconut sugar, honey, date paste, and monk fruit extract.

If you gradually reduce the amount of sugar you consume daily and how often you consume sugar, you will notice that you don't crave sweets as you used to. You will also notice that you gradually come to dislike the taste of highly sweetened foods (i.e., candies, cakes, pies, soft drinks, etc.). Finally, remember that your body has the ability to transform many substances into sugars—especially alcohols. Know that a large percentage of the alcohol that you intake is also being converted into sugars.

Drink as much water as possible so that you dilute the amount and concentrations of sugars in your body's tissues and organs. It should also be noted that higher sugar concentrations tend to lead to nerve and blood vessel damage too (because of the shape of the sugars and other reasons). So, if you desire to lose weight, to create a healthy lifestyle, and to avoid autoimmune conditions such as multiple sclerosis, then take control of your sugar intake. It will lead to a sweeter life.

Here are a few additional tips for reducing sugar intake and minimizing the impact of sugars on your mind and body:

- Use sugar-free preserves to sweeten plain yogurt, instead of eating already sweetened yogurt with fruit in it.
- Substitute healthy whole fruits for sweetened, processed desserts.
- Put fruit on your cereal instead of adding sugar or eating a sweetened cereal.
- Instead of a chocolate bar, have a lower-calorie, sugar-free hot chocolate drink.
- Snack on dried fruit or trail mix instead of candy.
- Buy unsweetened versions of applesauce, nut butters, nondairy milk, and other products that can hide added sugars.
- Add flavors such as vanilla, spices, or citrus to add a kick (and the illusion of sweetness) to your tea, coffee, and even oatmeal.[7]

---

[7] Sarah Stevenson, "10 Healthier Sugar Alternatives You Should Try," *Senior Living Blog: A Place for Mom*, February 17, 2015, https://www.aplaceformom.com/blog/2-17-15-healthy-sugar-alternatives/.

CHAPTER 3

Fats, Fatty Acids and Oils

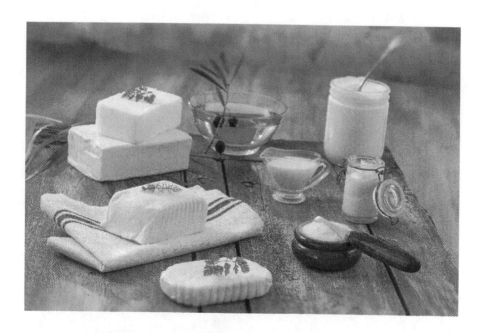

Fats and fat metabolism are next on the list. However, they could have easily been second on the list. The only reason sugars were covered before fats is because of the special roles that sugars tend to play in biochemical pathways and because of their roles in bodily communication with regard to metabolism.

However, it could easily be argued that fats also play very important roles in these processes. In any event, please don't discount the role of fats because the chapter dedicated to them follows the chapter on sugar. Fats are every bit as important, albeit in different ways. There's a reason why babies are born with a high fat content— so they can draw energy and warmth very quickly. In fact, babies specifically have a high content of brown fat as compared to children and adults.

According to Healthline,

> Each kind of fat serves a different purpose. White fat, or white adipose tissue (WAT), is the standard fat you've likely known about your whole life. It stores your energy in large fat droplets that accumulate around the body. The accumulation of fat helps keep you warm by literally providing insulation for your organs. In humans, too much white fat isn't a good thing. It leads to obesity. Too much white fat around the midsection may also create a higher risk of heart disease, diabetes, and other diseases. Brown fat, or brown adipose tissue (BAT), stores energy in a smaller space than white fat. It's packed with iron-rich mitochondria, which is how

it gets its color. When brown fat burns, it creates heat without shivering. This process is called thermogenesis. During this process, the brown fat also burns calories. Brown fat is highly regarded as a possible treatment for obesity and some metabolic syndromes. Scientists used to believe that only babies had brown fat, which makes up about 5 percent of their total body mass. They also thought this fat disappeared by the time most people reached adulthood. What researchers now know is that even adults have small reserves of brown fat. It's typically stored in small deposits around the shoulders and neck. In a way, brown fat is "good" fat. Humans with higher levels of brown fat may have lower bodyweights, for example. All people have some "constitutive" brown fat, which is the kind you're born with. There's also another form that's "recruitable." This means it can change to brown fat under the right circumstances. This recruitable type is found in muscles and white fat throughout your body. There are certain drugs that can cause the browning of white fat. Thiazolidinediones (TZDs), a drug used to help manage insulin resistance, can help with brown fat accumulation. However, this drug is also associated with weight gain, fluid retention, and other side effects. So, it can't be used as a quick fix for people looking to gain more brown fat. Exposing your body to cool and even cold temperatures may help recruit more brown fat cells. Some research has suggested that just two hours of exposure each day to temperatures around 66°F (19°C) may be enough to turn recruitable fat to brown. This fact might also help explain the physical appearance of certain geographical ethnic groups, in terms of fat distribution; such as the Eskimos.[8]

---

[8] Ashley Marcin, "Brown Fat: What You Should Know," Healthline, January 22, 2018, https://www.healthline.com/health/brown-fat#1.

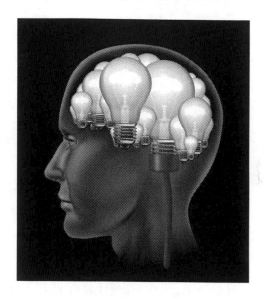

Fats have a plethora of purposes within the human body. Chief among these are the following:

- insulation
- energy production and storage
- transport
- biochemical communications (i.e., hormones)
- membrane structures.

According to the National Institutes of Health (NIH),

> When you have your cholesterol checked, the doctor typically gives you levels of three fats found in the blood: LDL, HDL and triglycerides. But did you know your body contains *thousands* of other types of fats, or lipids?

In human plasma alone, researchers have identified some 600 different types (of fats) relevant to our health. Many lipids are associated with diseases—diabetes, stroke, cancer, arthritis, Alzheimer's disease, to name a few. But our bodies also need a certain amount of fat to function, and we can't make it from scratch. Researchers funded by the National Institutes of Health are studying lipids to learn more about normal and abnormal biology. Triglycerides, cholesterol and other essential fatty acids—the scientific term for fats the body can't make on its own—store energy, insulate us and protect our vital organs. They act as messengers, helping proteins do their jobs. They also start biochemical reactions involved in growth, immune function, reproduction and other aspects of basic metabolism.

The cycle of making, breaking, storing and mobilizing fats is at the core of how humans and all animals regulate their energy. An imbalance in any step can result in disease, including heart disease and diabetes. For instance, having too many triglycerides in our bloodstream raises our risk of clogged arteries (i.e., arteriosclerosis and atherosclerosis), which can lead to heart attack and stroke.

Fats help the human body to stockpile certain nutrients as well. The "fat-soluble" vitamins—A, D, E and K—are stored in the liver and within other fatty tissues. Using a quantitative and systematic approach to study lipids, researchers have classified lipids into eight main categories. Cholesterol belongs to the "sterol" group, and triglycerides are "glycerolipids"; or glycolipids. Another category, "phospholipids," includes the hundreds of lipids that constitute our cell membranes and allow our cells and tissues to send and receive communication signals.

The main types of fat we consume, the *triglycerides*, are especially suited for energy storage; because they pack more than twice as much energy as carbohydrates or proteins. Once triglycerides have been broken down during digestion, then they are shipped out to cells throughout the bloodstream. Some of the fats also get utilized immediately for energy. The rest of the lipids are stored inside of cells; in blobs called lipid droplets. When we need extra energy—for instance, when we exercise (or have a fight or flight reaction)—then our bodies use enzymes called lipases to break down the stored triglycerides.

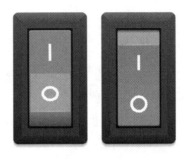

The cell's power plants, the mitochondria (which come only from your mother), can then create more of the body's main energy source: Adenosine Triphosphate (ATP). Recent research also has helped explain the functionality and purposes of a lipid called an omega-3 fatty acid—the active ingredient in cod liver oil; which has been touted for decades as a treatment for eczema, arthritis and heart diseases. Two types of these lipids blocked the activity of a protein called COX, which assists in converting an omega-6 fatty acid into pain-signaling prostaglandin molecules. These molecules are involved in inflammation, which is a common element of many diseases, so omega-3 fatty acids could have tremendous therapeutic potential.[9]

Earlier we stated that fats (i.e., lipids) have a plethora of purposes within the human body, including important roles in (1) insulation, (2) energy production and storage, (3) transport, (4) biochemical communications (by way of hormones), and (5) membrane structures. And these purposes underlie my chief opinions and recommendations regarding fat consumption and lipid lifestyle choices.

Generally, I recommend following a few general principles regarding fats that are fairly similar to those that I recommend regarding sugars:

- Do *not* eliminate cholesterol from you diet.
- Limit the types and amounts of fats you consume (when in doubt, look at the product label).
- Allow yourself to have cheat periods.
- Distinguish between saturated and unsaturated fats in your dietary choices (based on the product label).

---

[9]   NIH, National Institute of General Medical Sciences, "The Biology of Fats in the Body," *ScienceDaily*, April 23, 2013, www.sciencedaily.com/releases/2013/04/130423102127.htm.

- Choose natural fats over processed or engineered fats.
- Consume lots of water so that you can eliminate as much fat as possible through metabolism.
- Eat foods that are more fattening near the beginning of the day and leaner foods as the day progresses.
- Consume higher-fat-content foods in lower quantities.
- Finally, just as with sugars, if you gradually reduce the amount of fat you consume daily and the frequency with which you consume fatty foods, you will also notice that you don't crave fats as you used to. You will also notice that you gradually come to dislike the taste of highly fattening foods (e.g., rich creams and sauces, gravies).

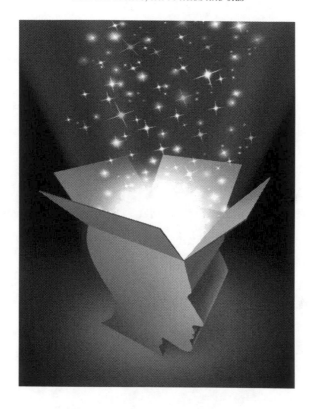

Remember that your body has the ability to transform many substances into adipose tissue—especially some sugars and carbohydrates. So, know that a large percentage of the carbohydrates that you intake will be converted into body fat. This means that you should watch the carbs! And remember, if your brain is chiefly made up of fats, then fats can't be all bad. Quantities matter almost as much as quality. It's the *balance* between quantities and quality that truly makes a real difference in diet.

Always know that the food product label is your ally in this process. All product labels clearly identify the types of fats in the product. Make sure that you pay close attention to the product label before you buy. It also helps if you buy your healthier groceries and products at places with more-knowledgeable employees—such as Sprouts, Whole Foods, and local health-oriented grocery stores and farmers markets. My advice is the same for every chapter of *The Nutrient Diet* that covers nutrition: don't ignore the product label.

CHAPTER 4

Carbohydrates and Ketones

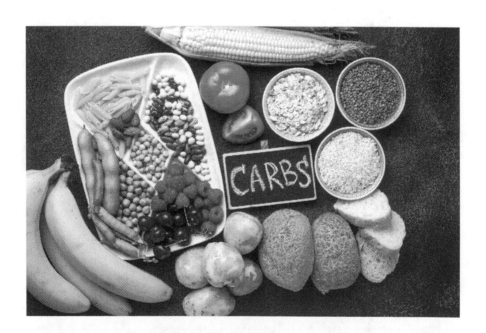

Carbohydrates and ketones could have been covered in either the chapter on sugars or the chapter on fats. However, since they have such a significant media presence (as with proteins and fats) right now, I decided to give them a full chapter of their very own. Carbohydrates and ketones have really gained the spotlight in recent years because of research that has been done in biochemistry and because of recent studies looking at paleo, keto, and Mediterranean diets. So, why are carbohydrates and ketones so important? Well, let's first talk about what they are.

Carbohydrates (carbon + H_2O) are basically long stacks of sugar molecules. They are generally placed into the following categories:

- sugars
- simple and complex carbohydrates
- resistant starch
- dietary fibers
- prebiotics
- intrinsic and added sugars.[10]

Biologically speaking, carbohydrates (i.e., carbon + water) are biological molecules containing carbon, hydrogen, and oxygen atoms in specific ratios. One of the primary functions of these carbohydrates is to provide your body with the energy it needs to complete its metabolic and biochemical processes. Most of the carbohydrates in the foods you consume get digested (beginning with salivary amylases) and are then broken down into glucose (the body's primary currency for sugar trading) before entering your bloodstream (by way

---

10   "The Functions of Carbohydrates in the Body," EUFIC, January 14, 2020, https://www.eufic.org/en/whats-in-food/article/the-basics-carbohydrates.

of arteries and arterioles [i.e., small arteries]). Glucose in the bloodstream is normally taken up into somatic cells and used to produce the body's most efficient fuel molecule, adenosine triphosphate (ATP, the body's primary currency for energy trading), through a series of complex processes and biochemical steps known collectively as cellular respiration. These somatic cells then use ATP to power a plethora of metabolic tasks at both the cellular and tissue level. Most cells in the body (i.e., somatic cells) are quite capable of producing ATP from several different sources, including dietary carbohydrates and lipids. However, if you are continually consuming a diet with a combination of these molecular substances, then the vast majority of your somatic cells will gradually learn and evolve to prefer to use carbohydrates as their chief energy source.

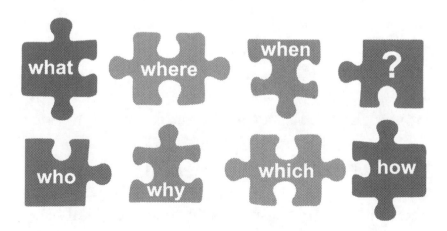

When your body has enough glucose to fulfill its present requirements, any excess glucose quantities are stored for use in future activities. This stored form of glucose is called glycogen. Glycogen is chiefly stored in tissues such as the liver and in skeletal muscles (so that it can be quickly mobilized if needed immediately). These stored glucose molecules are able to be released into the bloodstream to provide energy to somatic cells and to consistently maintain a normal range of blood sugar levels during the fasting state, that is, between meals.

However, unlike the glycogen molecules stored within the liver, the glycogen that is stored within skeletal muscles can only be used by other muscle cells (i.e., they are muscle-specific). Therefore, it is essential during long periods of high-intensity muscular activity, such as lifting weights, doing aerobic exercise, running, or walking briskly. Furthermore, when all your somatic cells have all the glucose they require and your glycogen stores are full, your body will convert these excess carbohydrates into triglyceride molecules, storing them as fat in lipocytes.

Glycogen storage is simply one of multiple methods that your body's tissues and organs employ to ensure they have an adequate supply of glucose (i.e., energy) for their vital functions and biochemical processes.

When glucose from carbohydrate sources falls short, skeletal muscle cells and tissues can also be broken down into amino acids and converted into glucose or other compounds to generate energy. Obviously, this isn't an ideal scenario since muscle cells are crucial for body movement, which is a basic bodily function. In severe instances, such as during famine, when individuals develop conditions such as Kwashiorkor or Marasmus, this can lead to death. However, this is one reliable method that the human body has developed to ensure adequate energy supplies for the brain, a method that requires a reserve of energy (from glucose) during periods of prolonged starvation. Therefore, consuming at least a small quantity carbohydrates in the diet daily is one method of proactively preventing starvation-related loss of body muscle mass. These carbohydrates will also reduce the degree of muscle breakdown while providing enough glucose to the brain for its important activities.[11]

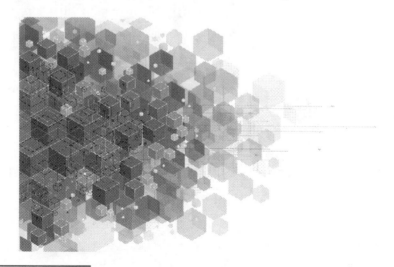

[11]   D. G. Sapir, O. E. Owen, J. T. Cheng, R. Ginsberg, G. Boden, and W. G. Walker, "The Effect of Carbohydrates on Ammonium and Ketoacid Excretion during Starvation," *Journal of Clinical Investigation* 51, no. 8 (1972): 2093–2102, https://doi.org/10.1172/JCI107016, retrieved from https://www.ncbi.nlm.nih.gov/pmc/articles/PMC292366/.

Unlike sugars and starches, dietary fiber, another form of carbohydrate, is not reduced to glucose. Instead, it passes through the body largely undigested. At that point, it is categorized as one of two primary types of fiber: (1) soluble fiber and (2) insoluble fiber. The soluble form of fiber is found within oats and within the inner portions of many fruits and vegetables. Additionally, during digestion and other metabolic and biochemical activities, the soluble form of fiber draws in water (i.e., it is hydrophilic) to form a gelatinous substance. This gelatinous substance causes an increase in the bulk of the stool, softening it in order to make bowel movements less uncomfortable (i.e., less damaging to the rectum and anus). Specifically, in a review of several placebo-controlled studies, soluble forms of fiber were found to improve the consistency of stools and to raise the frequency of bowel movements in patients with constipation. Consequently, higher consumption levels of soluble fiber will significantly reduce the degree of straining and pain associated with producing bowel movements, which also prevents hemorrhoid conditions and hematochezia.[12]

---

[12] N. C. Suares and A. C. Ford, "Systematic Review: The Effects of Fibre in the Management of Chronic Idiopathic Constipation," *Alimentary Pharmacology & Therapeutics* 33, no. 8 (2011): 895–901, https://doi.org/10.1111/j.1365-2036.2011.04602.x, retrieved from https://pubmed.ncbi.nlm.nih.gov/21332763/.

By contrast, the more insoluble forms of fiber, that is, the forms that do not draw in water, help to prevent and alleviate constipation by adding bulk to stools and by speeding up the velocity with which they move through the digestive tract. This more insoluble form of fiber is found in whole grains. It is also found within the skins and seeds of both vegetables and fruits.

Finally, obtaining an adequate daily quantity of insoluble fiber will protect against a host of other digestive tract diseases. Specifically, a particular observational study of approximately forty thousand men found that higher levels of intake of insoluble forms of fiber led to a greater than 30 percent reduction in risk for diverticular diseases, a group of conditions in which thin, fragile pouches develop in the intestine as a result of regular straining during bowel movements. Obviously, eating excessive quantities of processed and refined carbohydrates is not particularly beneficial to your heart and other organs. It could lead to an increase in your risk of developing type 2 diabetes. However, regularly consuming and utilizing adequate quantities of soluble and insoluble forms of dietary fiber will benefit your heart while helping to sustain blood glucose concentration levels within the normal range.[13]

---

[13] S. Liu, W. C. Willett, M. J. Stampfer, et al., "A Prospective Study of Dietary Glycemic Load, Carbohydrate Intake, and Risk of Coronary Heart Disease in US Women," *American Journal of Clinical Nutrition* 71, no. 6 (2000): 1455–61, https://doi.org/10.1093/ajcn/71.6.1455, retrieved

When soluble fiber passes through certain portions of the small intestines, it will bind with bile acids to prevent from being reabsorbed by the intestines. However, in order to manufacture additional bile acids, the liver has to utilize cholesterol, which normally would simply travel through the bloodstream. Several placebo-controlled studies have illustrated that taking approximately ten grams of psyllium (a supplement of soluble fiber) daily can decrease the percentage of low LDL (i.e., the so-called bad cholesterol) cholesterol by approximately 7 percent. Furthermore, a cursory review of over twenty different observational studies showed a 9 percent decreased risk for heart disease with every additional seven grams of soluble dietary fiber consumed daily. Note that fiber does not raise blood glucose levels in the way that other carbohydrates do. To the contrary, soluble fiber helps to delay the absorption of complex carbohydrates in the digestive tract, leading to even lower blood sugar levels during the fasting state.[14]

---

from https://www.ncbi.nlm.nih.gov/pubmed/18039988; A. W. Barclay, P. Petocz, J. McMillan-Price, et al., "Glycemic Index, Glycemic Load, and Chronic Disease Risk—a Meta-Analysis of Observational Studies," *American Journal of Clinical Nutrition* 87, no. 3 (2008): 627–37, https://doi.org/10.1093/ajcn/87.3.627, retrieved from https://www.ncbi.nlm.nih.gov/pubmed/18326601.

[14] S. M. Tosh, "Review of Human Studies Investigating the Post-Prandial Blood-Glucose-Lowering Ability of Oat and Barley Food Products," *European Journal of Clinical Nutrition* 67, no. 4 (April 2013): 310–17, https://

A review of over thirty studies illustrated significant reductions in fasting blood glucose levels when patients took soluble fiber supplements on a daily basis, leading to even lower hemoglobin A1c levels in diabetic patients. Correlatively, although the consumption of soluble fiber did decrease the blood glucose levels in patients categorized as prediabetic, it was the most efficacious (i.e., clinically potent and significant) in patients struggling to manage a diagnosis of type 2 diabetes.[15]

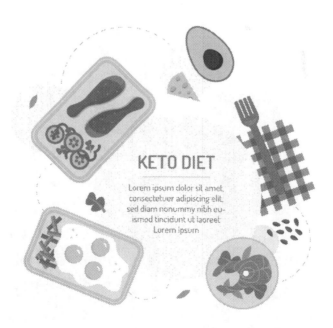

KETO DIET

Lorem ipsum dolor sit amet, consectetuer adipiscing elit, sed diam nonummy nibh euismod tincidunt ut laoreet Lorem ipsum

doi.org/10.1038/ejcn.2013.25, retrieved from https://pubmed.ncbi.nlm.nih. gov/23422921/.

[15]   Keith Pearson, "What Are the Key Functions of Carbohydrates?" Healthline,   November   9,   2017,   https://www.healthline. com/nutrition/carbohydrate-functions.

Now, what about ketones? First of all, ketosis is a natural human metabolic and biochemical state of being. As such, it involves the body's processes for producing ketone bodies from fat molecules and then utilizing them for energy (instead of using carbohydrates). You can easily get into a state of metabolic ketosis by following a low-carbohydrate, fat-rich (i.e., ketogenic) diet. In addition to the physical advantage of quick loss of weight (especially fatty tissues), ketosis also offers numerous other health benefits, including the recognized ability to decrease the quality and quantity of seizure activity in epileptic children.[16]

Ketosis is a highly complex biological and metabolic process, but it's essentially a metabolic and biochemical state in which fat provides the vast majority of the fuel for the body's activities. Ketosis occurs when there is limited access to plasma glucose, which is the more preferred fuel source for a plethora of tissues and cells within the body. Ketosis is quite often associated with ketogenic diets, which are very low in carbohydrates. Ketosis also happens during pregnancy, infancy, fasting,

---

[16] R. G. Levy, P. N. Cooper, and P. Giri, "Ketogenic Diet and Other Dietary Treatments for Epilepsy," *Cochrane Database of Systematic Reviews* 3 (March 14, 2012): CD001903, https://doi.org/10.1002/14651858.CD001903.pub2, retrieved from https://www.ncbi.nlm.nih.gov/pubmed/22419282.

and starvation—states characterized by an increased need for metabolic energy supplies.[17]

To go into ketosis, people generally need to consume less than fifty grams of carbs per day, and sometimes as little as twenty grams per day. This circumstance requires the removal of certain food items from the daily diet, such as grains, candies, soft drinks, and sweetened fruit juices (especially those containing high-fructose corn syrup). These types of dieters will also need to cut back on potatoes, fruits, and other foods that have a high concentration of starches. When one is consuming a diet that is low in carbohydrate concentrations, the level of the metabolic hormone insulin decreases and fatty

---

[17]   P. Y. Wu, J. Edmond, N. Auestad, S. Rambathla, J. Benson, and T. Picone, "Medium-Chain Triglycerides in Infant Formulas and Their Relation to Plasma Ketone Body Concentrations," *Pediatric Research* 20, no. 4 (1986): 338–41, https://doi.org/10.1203/00006450-198604000-00016, https://www.ncbi.nlm.nih.gov/pubmed/3703623; S. C. Cunnane and M. A. Crawford, "Survival of the Fattest: Fat Babies Were the Key to Evolution of the Large Human Brain," *Comparative Biochemistry and Physiology Part A, Molecular & Integrative Physiology* 136, no. 1 (2003): 17–26, https://doi.org/10.1016/s1095-6433(03)00048-5, retrieved from https://www.ncbi.nlm.nih.gov/pubmed/14527626; T. Fukao, G. D. Lopaschuk, and G. A. Mitchell, "Pathways and Control of Ketone Body Metabolism: On the Fringe of Lipid Biochemistry," *Prostaglandins, Leukotrines, & Essential Fatty Acids* 70, no. 3 (2004): 243–51, https://doi.org/10.1016/j.plefa.2003.11.001, retrieved from https://www.ncbi.nlm.nih.gov/pubmed/14769483; O. E. Owen, P. Felig, A. P. Morgan, J. Wahren, and G. F. Cahill Jr., "Liver and Kidney Metabolism during Prolonged Starvation," *Journal of Clinical Investigation* 48, no. 3 (1969): 574–83, https://doi.org/10.1172/JCI106016, retrieved from https://www.ncbi.nlm.nih.gov/pubmed/5773093/.

acids are released from the body's fat stores in much greater quantities, leading to a higher degree of quick weight loss. Great quantities of these fatty acids are then transferred to the liver, where they are oxidized and metabolically (i.e., biochemically) transformed into ketones (i.e., ketone bodies). These ketone bodies, much like glucose, are able to provide energy for the entire body. However, unlike most fatty acids, ketones can also be transported across the blood-brain barrier (i.e., the barrier created by the brain to selectively allow some molecules and substances to pass through while blocking the transport of others) and then provide energy for the brain when glucose is unavailable.

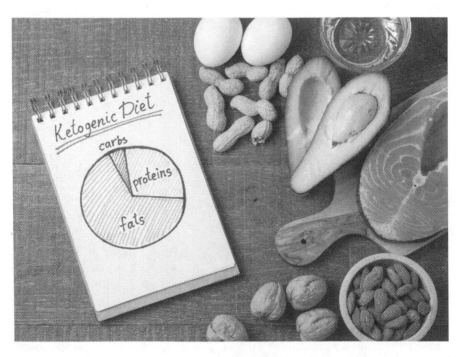

It's a common misconception that the human brain cannot properly function without the use of dietary carbohydrates. Nevertheless, it is factual that the brain normally prefers to use glucose and that some brain tissues, regions and areas can only use glucose for fuel. However, a vast geographic portion of the human brain can also easily utilize ketone bodies as an energy source. This may be the case in a state of starvation or when the availability of carbohydrates is limited.[18]

For instance, after only three days of starvation, the brain will begin to draw as much as 25 percent of its energy from ketone bodies. And during periods of long-term starvation, the brain will draw as much as 60 percent (i.e., two-thirds) of its energy from ketone bodies. Furthermore, the human body can also utilize protein (in the form of amino acids) in order to produce the additional glucose the brain may require during ketosis. This metabolic process is called gluconeogenesis, which is a cornerstone of human biochemistry.[19]

---

[18] J. C. LaManna, N. Salem, M. Puchowicz, et al., "Ketones Suppress Brain Glucose Consumption," *Advances in Experimental Medicine and Biology* 645 (2009): 301–6, https://doi.org/10.1007/978-0-387-85998-9_45, retrieved from https://www.ncbi.nlm.nih.gov/pubmed/19227486/.

[19] S. G. Hasselbalch, G. M. Knudsen, J. Jakobsen, L. P. Hageman, S. Holm, and O. B. Paulson, "Brain Metabolism during Short-Term Starvation in Humans," *Journal of Cerebral Blood Flow and Metabolism* 14, no. 1 (1994): 125–31, https://doi.org/10.1038/jcbfm.1994.17, retrieved from https://www.ncbi.nlm.nih.gov/pubmed/8263048/; O. E. Owen, A. P. Morgan, H. G. Kemp, J. M. Sullivan, M. G. Herrera, and G. F. Cahill Jr., "Brain Metabolism

Correspondingly, together, ketosis and gluconeogenesis are capable of satisfying all the brain's energy requirements on a daily basis. However, a great number of people continue to confuse the process of ketosis with the metabolic disorder known as ketoacidosis. Moreover, while ketosis is a normal (and relatively health-sustaining) metabolic process, ketoacidosis, by contrast, is an adverse metabolic condition that can lead to coma and even death if not treated promptly. In the ketoacidotic state, the bloodstream is saturated with fastidious concentrations of both glucose and ketones. As a direct consequence, the blood becomes unsustainably and dangerously acidic, which is directly detrimental to cells, tissues, organs, organelles, and cellular respiration. Specifically, ketoacidosis is generally seen in patients with type 1 diabetes that is chronically uncontrolled (i.e., mismanaged). In addition, it can occur in people with type 2 diabetes, although this is not nearly as common in these patients since their pancreatic beta cells do still possess some level of insulin production. Finally, severe alcohol abuse commonly leads to ketoacidosis.[20]

---

during Fasting," *Journal of Clinical Investigation* 46, no. 10 (1967): 1589–95, https://doi.org/10.1172/JCI105650, retrieved from https://www.ncbi.nlm.nih.gov/pubmed/6061736/.

[20] A. R. Gosmanov, E. O. Gosmanova, and E. Dillard-Cannon, "Management of Adult Diabetic Ketoacidosis," *Diabetes, Metabolic Syndrome, and Obesity* 7 (June 30, 2014): 255–64, https://doi.org/10.2147/DMSO.S50516, retrieved from https://www.ncbi.nlm.nih.gov/

Let's take a look at the role of ketones and ketosis in the specialty of neurology. Epilepsy is a neurological disorder characterized by the presence of recurring seizures. It's a common neurological condition from which approximately seventy million people suffer in one form or another worldwide. Thankfully for most patients, readily available antiseizure medications are able to manage and control the vast majority of their seizures. However, unfortunately, for a plethora of reasons, approximately 30 percent of epileptic patients fail standard therapies and continue to experience seizures regularly despite the wide availability and long track records of these antiseizure medications. Interestingly enough, during the 1920s, a revolutionary ketogenic diet was first introduced to treat patients with epilepsy who had failed with common therapies (i.e., they suffered from a drug-resistant form of epilepsy). The ketogenic diet has typically been used in children with epilepsy and other disorders marked by seizures, and several studies have revealed remarkable outcomes using the ketogenic approach to seizure prevention, management, and control. For instance, a large number of children and adolescents suffering from seizures have experience highly clinically significant reductions

---

pubmed/25061324/; L. C. McGuire, A. M. Cruickshank, and P. T. Munro, "Alcoholic Ketoacidosis," *Emergency Medicine Journal* 23, no. 6 (2006): 417–20, https://doi.org/10.1136/emj.2004.017590, retrieved from https://www.ncbi.nlm.nih.gov/pubmed/16714496.

in the number of seizures and the degree of seizure activity while being on the ketogenic diet, and some of them have experienced the complete remission of epileptic activity.[21]

Moreover, the ketogenic diet is a data-driven strategy with regard to weight management and seizure control fairly well supported by scientific research and clinical trial data. For example, some clinical trials and studies have revealed that people who follow ketogenic diets tend to experience a greater loss of weight (and, hence, fatty tissue) at a faster rate than those who follow other popular low-fat diets and weight-management approaches.[22]

---

[21]   J. M. Freeman, E. P. Vining, D. J. Pillas, P. L. Pyzik, J. C. Casey, and L. M. Kelly, "The Efficacy of the Ketogenic Diet—1998: A Prospective Evaluation of Intervention in 150 Children," *Pediatrics* 102, no. 6 (1998): 1358–63, https://doi.org/10.1542/peds.102.6.1358, retrieved from https://www.ncbi. nlm.nih.gov/pubmed/9832569; H. C. Kang, Y. J. Kim, D. W. Kim, and H. D. Kim, "Efficacy and Safety of the Ketogenic Diet for Intractable Childhood Epilepsy: Korean Multicentric Experience," *Epilepsia* 46, no. 2 (2005): 272–79, https://doi.org/10.1111/j.0013-9580.2005.48504.x, retrieved from https://www.ncbi.nlm.nih.gov/pubmed/15679508; E. G. Neal, H. Chaffe, R. H. Schwartz, et al., "The Ketogenic Diet for the Treatment of Childhood Epilepsy: A Randomised Controlled Trial," *Lancet Neurology* 7, no. 6 (2008): 500–6, https://doi.org/10.1016/S1474-4422(08)70092-9, retrieved from https://www.ncbi.nlm.nih.gov/pubmed/18456557; H. F. Li, Y. Zou, and G. Ding, "Therapeutic Success of the Ketogenic Diet as a Treatment Option for Epilepsy: A Meta-Analysis," *Iranian Journal of Pediatrics* 23, no. 6 (2013): 613–20, https://www.ncbi.nlm.nih.gov/pubmed/24910737.
[22]   W. S. Yancy Jr., M. K. Olsen, J. R. Guyton, R. P. Bakst, and E. C. Westman, "A Low-Carbohydrate, Ketogenic Diet versus a Low-Fat Diet to Treat Obesity and Hyperlipidemia: A Randomized, Controlled

One particularly robust study found that ketogenic diet patients lost twice as much weight within the same period compared to their counterparts being treated with a low-fat, calorie-restricted diet.[23] Furthermore, individuals have reported that they tend to feel less hungry (and, hence, more satiated) on a ketogenic diet, which scientists have attributed to a positive effect of ketosis/ketogenesis. Therefore, ketogenic diet participants have found it unnecessary to count calories while on the diet.[24]

Trial," *Annals of Internal Medicine* 140, no. 10 (2004): 769–77, https://doi.org/10.7326/0003-4819-140-10-200405180-00006, retrieved from https://www.ncbi.nlm.nih.gov/pubmed/15148063; L. Stern, N. Iqbal, P. Seshadri, et al., "The Effects of Low-Carbohydrate versus Conventional Weight Loss Diets in Severely Obese Adults: One-Year Follow-Up of a Randomized Trial," *Annals of Internal Medicine* 140, no. 10 (2004): 778–85, https://doi.org/10.7326/0003-4819-140-10-200405180-00007, retrieved from https://www.ncbi.nlm.nih.gov/pubmed/15148064; J. Volek, M. Sharman, A. Gómez A, et al., "Comparison of Energy-Restricted Very Low-Carbohydrate and Low-Fat Diets on Weight Loss and Body Composition in Overweight Men and Women," *Nutrition & Metabolism* (London) 1, no. 1 (November 8, 2004): 13, https://doi.org/10.1186/1743-7075-1-13, retrieved from https://www.ncbi.nlm.nih.gov/pubmed/15533250/.

[23] B. J. Brehm, R. J. Seeley, S. R. Daniels, and D. A. D'Alessio, "A Randomized Trial Comparing a Very Low-Carbohydrate Diet and a Calorie-Restricted Low-Fat Diet on Body Weight and Cardiovascular Risk Factors in Healthy Women," *Journal of Clinical Endocrinology and Metabolism* 88, no. 4 (2003): 1617–23, https://doi.org/10.1210/jc.2002-021480, retrieved from https://www.ncbi.nlm.nih.gov/pubmed/12679447.

[24] A. A. Gibson, R. V. Seimon, C. M. Lee, et al., "Do Ketogenic Diets Really Suppress Appetite? A Systematic Review and Meta-Analysis," *Obesity Reviews* 16, no. 1 (2015): 64–76, https://doi.org/10.1111/obr.12230, retrieved from https://www.ncbi.nlm.nih.gov/pubmed/25402637; F. J. McClernon, W. S. Yancy Jr., J. A. Eberstein, R. C. Atkins, and E. C. Westman, "The

Ketosis and ketogenic diets also have other therapeutic effects on metabolism and bodily fuel utilization and management processes. In fact, ketogenic approaches are now being researched and considered for treatments and adjunctive therapies for a wide host of additional medical conditions,[25] including the following:

- Heart disease
  Reducing carbs to achieve ketosis may improve heart disease risk factors such as blood triglycerides, total cholesterol, and HDL cholesterol.[26]

- Type 2 diabetes

Effects of a Low-Carbohydrate Ketogenic Diet and a Low-Fat Diet on Mood, Hunger, and Other Self-Reported Symptoms," *Obesity* (Silver Spring) 15, no. 1 (2007): 182–87, https://doi.org/10.1038/oby.2007.516, retrieved from https://www.ncbi.nlm.nih.gov/pubmed/17228046.

[25] A. Paoli, A. Rubini, J. S. Volek, and K. A. Grimaldi, "Beyond Weight Loss: A Review of the Therapeutic Uses of Very Low-Carbohydrate (Ketogenic) Diets" [published correction appears in *European Journal of Clinical Nutrition* 68, no. 5 (May 2014): 641], *European Journal of Clinical Nutrition* 67, no. 8 (2013): 789–96, https://doi.org/10.1038/ejcn.2013.116, retrieved from https://www.ncbi.nlm.nih.gov/pubmed/23801097/.

[26] M. J. Sharman, W. J. Kraemer, D. M. Love, et al., "A Ketogenic Diet Favorably Affects Serum Biomarkers for Cardiovascular Disease in Normal-Weight Men," *Journal of Nutrition* 132, no. 7 (2002): 1879–85, https://doi.org/10.1093/jn/132.7.1879, retrieved from https://www.ncbi.nlm.nih.gov/pubmed/12097663/; J. S. Volek, M. J. Sharman, and C. E. Forsythe, "Modification of Lipoproteins by Very Low-Carbohydrate Diets," *Journal of Nutrition* 135, no. 6 (2005): 1339–42, https://doi.org/10.1093/jn/135.6.1339, retrieved from https://www.ncbi.nlm.nih.gov/pubmed/15930434/.

The diet may improve insulin sensitivity by up to 75 percent, with some diabetics being able to reduce or even stop diabetes medication.[27]

- Metabolic syndrome
Ketogenic diets can improve all major symptoms of metabolic syndrome, including high triglycerides, excess belly fat, and elevated blood pressure.[28]

- Alzheimer's disease
A ketogenic diet may have benefits for patients with Alzheimer's disease.[29]

---

[27]   G. Boden, K. Sargrad, C. Homko, M. Mozzoli, and T. P. Stein, "Effect of a Low-Carbohydrate Diet on Appetite, Blood Glucose Levels, and Insulin Resistance in Obese Patients with Type 2 Diabetes," *Annals of Internal Medicine* 142, no. 6 (2005): 403–11, https://doi.org/10.7326/0003-4819-142-6-200503150-00006, retrieved from https://www.ncbi.nlm.nih.gov/pubmed/15767618; E. C. Westman, W. S. Yancy Jr., J. C. Mavropoulos, M. Marquart, and J. R. McDuffie, "The Effect of a Low-Carbohydrate, Ketogenic Diet versus a Low-Glycemic Index Diet on Glycemic Control in Type 2 Diabetes Mellitus," *Nutrition & Metabolism* (London) 5 (December 19, 2008): 36, https://doi.org/10.1186/1743-7075-5-36, retrieved from https://www.ncbi.nlm.nih.gov/pubmed/19099589/.

[28]   R. D. Feinman and M. Makowske, "Metabolic Syndrome and Low-Carbohydrate Ketogenic Diets in the Medical School Biochemistry Curriculum," *Metabolic Syndrome and Related Disorders* 1, no. 3 (2003): 189–97, https://doi.org/10.1089/154041903322716660, retrieved from https://www.ncbi.nlm.nih.gov/pubmed/18370662.

[29]   S. T. Henderson, J. L. Vogel, L. J. Barr, F. Garvin, J. J. Jones, and L. C. Costantini, "Study of the Ketogenic Agent AC-1202 in Mild to Moderate Alzheimer's Disease: A Randomized, Double-Blind, Placebo-Controlled, Multicenter Trial," *Nutrition & Metabolism* (London) 6 (August 10, 2009):

- Cancer
Some studies suggest that ketogenic diets may aid in cancer therapy, possibly by helping to "starve" cancer cells of glucose.[30]

- Parkinson's disease
A small study found that symptoms of Parkinson's disease improved after twenty-eight days on a ketogenic diet.[31]

- Acne
There is some evidence that this diet may reduce the severity and progression of acne.[32]

31, https://doi.org/10.1186/1743-7075-6-31, retrieved from https://www.ncbi.nlm.nih.gov/pubmed/19664276/.

[30] E. J. Fine, C. J. Segal-Isaacson, R. D. Feinman, et al., "Targeting Insulin Inhibition as a Metabolic Therapy in Advanced Cancer: A Pilot Safety and Feasibility Dietary Trial in 10 Patients," *Nutrition* 28, no. 10 (2012): 1028–35, https://doi.org/10.1016/j.nut.2012.05.001, retrieved from https://www.ncbi.nlm.nih.gov/pubmed/22840388/; W. Zhou, P. Mukherjee, M. A. Kiebish, W. T. Markis, J. G. Mantis, and T. N. Seyfried, "The Calorically Restricted Ketogenic Diet, an Effective Alternative Therapy for Malignant Brain Cancer," *Nutrition & Metabolism* (London) 4 (February 21, 2007): 5; https://doi.org/10.1186/1743-7075-4-5, retrieved from https://www.ncbi.nlm.nih.gov/pubmed/17313687/.

[31] T. B. Vanitallie, C. Nonas, A. Di Rocco, K. Boyar, K. Hyams, and S. B. Heymsfield, "Treatment of Parkinson Disease with Diet-Induced Hyperketonemia: A Feasibility Study," *Neurology* 64, no. 4 (2005): 728–30, https://doi.org/10.1212/01.WNL.0000152046.11390.45, retrieved from https://www.ncbi.nlm.nih.gov/pubmed/15728303/.

[32] A. Paoli, K. Grimaldi, L. Toniolo, M. Canato, A. Bianco, A. Fratter, "Nutrition and Acne: Therapeutic Potential of Ketogenic Diets," *Skin Pharmacology and Physiology* 25, no. 3 (2012): 111–17, https://doi.

However, ketosis and ketogenic diets are not without side effects and potential disadvantages. Some of the more commonly reported side effects include headaches, fatigue and lethargy, constipation, hyperlipidemia (high cholesterol levels), and malodorous breath.[33]

However, it has been reported that many of these symptoms are temporary in nature, often disappearing within days or weeks. In addition, some children on ketogenic diets have reported the appearance and persistence of kidney stones.[34]

---

org/10.1159/000336404, retrieved from https://www.ncbi.nlm.nih.gov/pubmed/22327146.

[33] C. Wibisono, N. Rowe, E. Beavis, et al., "Ten-Year Single-Center Experience of the Ketogenic Diet: Factors Influencing Efficacy, Tolerability, and Compliance," *Journal of Pediatrics* 166, no. 4 (2015): 1030–36.e1, https://doi.org/10.1016/j.jpeds.2014.12.018, retrieved from https://www.ncbi.nlm.nih.gov/pubmed/25649120; G. R. Zamani, M. Mohammadi, M. R. Ashrafi, et al., "The Effects of Classic Ketogenic Diet on Serum Lipid Profile in Children with Refractory Seizures," *Acta Neurologica Belgica* 116, no. 4 (2016): 529–34, https://doi.org/10.1007/s13760-016-0601-x, retrieved from https://www.ncbi.nlm.nih.gov/pubmed/26791878.

[34] A. Sampath, E. H. Kossoff, S. L. Furth, P. L. Pyzik, and E. P. Vining, "Kidney Stones and the Ketogenic Diet: Risk Factors and Prevention," *Journal of Child Neurology* 22, no. 4 (2007): 375–78, https://doi.org/10.1177/0883073807301926, retrieved from https://www.ncbi.nlm.nih.gov/pubmed/17621514; S. Kielb, H. P. Koo, D. A. Bloom, and G. J. Faerber, "Nephrolithiasis Associated with the Ketogenic Diet," *Journal of Urology* 164, no. 2 (200): 464–66, https://www.ncbi.nlm.nih.gov/pubmed/10893623; S. L. Furth, J. C. Casey, P. L. Pyzik, et al., "Risk Factors for Urolithiasis in Children on the Ketogenic Diet," *Pediatric Nephrology* 15, no. 1–2 (2000): 125–28, https://doi.org/10.1007/s004670000443, retrieved from https://www.ncbi.nlm.nih.gov/pubmed/11095028.

Individuals being treated with agents used to address diabetes should consult with their primary care physicians prior to attempting a ketogenic diet, since a ketogenic diet could alter their need for medication. Furthermore, some ketogenic approaches are characterized by lowered levels of consumption of fiber. Because of this, beginners of a ketogenic diet may want to supplement the diet with high-fiber, low-carb vegetables, at least in the beginning, until the body has a chance to get used to the new diet. Nonetheless, ketosis is generally safe for most individuals who lack an underlying health condition. Still, the ketogenic diet is not the best choice for everyone. Notably, some individuals will feel a renewed sense of energy while on the diet, while others may feel depressed, lethargic, tired, or exhausted.[35]

So, what are the take-home points for carbohydrates and ketones (i.e., ketone bodies)? Well, there are many! First, I would recommend that you consider the percentages of carbohydrates and fiber within your daily nutrient intake. Balance and proportion definitely matter. Try to ingest the recommended amount of carbohydrates each day. Also, if possible, take in most of your carbohydrates during the earlier, more active parts of the day. In furtherance of this goal, I would

---

[35] Hrefna Palsdottir, "What Is Ketosis, and Is It Healthy?" June 3, 2017, Healthline, https://www.healthline.com/nutrition/what-is-ketosis.

recommend that you lower the percentages of carbs that you intake as the day progresses so that by four o'clock in the afternoon you have consumed 80 percent of your daily carbohydrates.

I would also recommend that you gradually increase your fiber intake as the day progresses in just the opposite way in which you deal with carbohydrates. As the day progresses, your intake of carbohydrates, sweets, and fats should decrease as your intake of proteins, vegetables, and fiber sources increases. I would also recommend that you limit the percentage of processed and/or modified carbohydrates you consume, or eliminate these altogether. In general, the less processed your carbohydrates, the better. The same goes for fats and proteins. The consumption of high percentages of genetically modified, genetically engineered, highly processed, and/or artificial foods may promote the development of autoimmune symptoms, conditions, and/or disorders. Also, if possible, if and when you consume carbohydrates that have been exposed to oils, use healthier oils such as coconut oil, rather than less healthy oils such as olive oil or highly processed margarine. As far as ketones go, I would advise caution regarding the use of a ketogenic diet.

While there are benefits to the adoption or partial adoption of a ketogenic diet, quite a few risks exist by following such a diet. I would strongly recommend that you only undertake a ketogenic diet under the guidance and supervision of your primary care physician or another similarly trained physician. Obviously, patients suffering from epilepsy or other diseases marked by seizures should consult with both their primary care physician and a neurologist when considering using a ketogenic approach to seizure management and control. However, regardless of weight loss goals and/or neurological goals, I would strongly recommend against the regular consumption of drinks and/or foodstuffs that contain high percentages of high-fructose corn syrup. As cited earlier, to go into ketosis, people generally need to consume fewer than fifty grams of carbs per day, and sometimes as little as twenty grams per day. This circumstance requires the removal of certain food items from the daily diet, such as grains, candies, soft drinks, and sweetened fruit juices (especially those containing high-fructose corn syrup). These types of dieters will also need to cut back on potatoes, fruits, and other foods that have a high concentration of starches. Therefore, I generally recommend the limitation or full elimination of soft drinks and drinks containing high-fructose corn syrup from your diet. Finally, I recommend a ketogenic approach because it will deeply limit your risk of developing diabetes. As discussed in the first chapter, a larger dietary consumption of water will also help in this regard.

If you're truly interested in trying a ketogenic diet, I would recommend that you go straight to the experts. Check out the studies, research, papers, and presentations by experts such as Dr. Christopher M. Palmer. Dr. Palmer has been using the ketogenic diet at his practices for over fifteen years now. He is the director of the Department of Postgraduate and Continuing Education at McLean Hospital and an assistant professor of psychiatry at Harvard Medical School. Given that he is the definitive expert on the ketogenic diet, his papers, presentations, and other research will show you the metabolic and biochemical pathways affected by a ketogenic diet. You don't have to understand everything about it, but you should make an effort to understand the risks, side effects, pros, cons, complications, and overall picture before you try it.

CHAPTER 5

Proteins, Enzymes, and Amino Acids

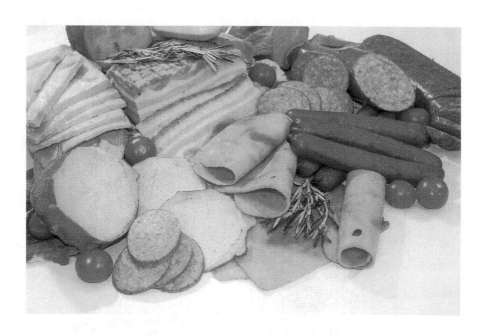

Proteins are required in our diets. Essentially, proteins are needed for the amino acids that they contain and into which they can be broken down. Proteins, just like sugars and fats, can be simple, complex, or anything in between. And, just like sugars, fats and other biochemical substances (such as neurotransmitters), proteins are vastly recycled throughout our tissues and organs. They are an integral part of energy transfers and cellular respiration and communication. They are also central to the viability of human life and the ability of humans to survive and be ecologically successful. In addition, amino acids are combined into groupings that form "bases." These bases are used as currency in quite a few biochemical operations, including the storage of genetic material. The foundation and basis of our ability to pass on genetic potential (genes generally code for proteins) and complete the necessary biological and biochemical processes needed for survival is proteins. Amino acids and proteins are also extremely vital to the communication between cells, tissues, organs, and organ systems. Given this fact, I would consider amino acids and proteins to be every bit as important to healthy human life as sugars (used by the body to produce energy) and fats (used by the body to make hormones). Therefore, they definitely deserve our full attention.

Just as is the case with both sugars and fats, our bodies have to the ability to interchange amino acids and proteins and transform them from one form to another. In this way, they are used for energy use, energy storage, and communication. They are currency and energy, just like sugars and fats. However, in our daily lives, we tend to prefer that our bodies convert currencies into more compact storage forms—just as our DNA does with genetic instructions. DNA is just a complex condensed form of genetic storage for the language of human life and development. As books such as *The Biology of Belief* by Dr. Bruce H. Lipton explain, genes are only as important as their ability to be turned on. Because of this, the best genes in the world mean absolutely nothing in environments where they will never be turned on (such as a plant placed in complete darkness)—just as the most advanced computer in the world would be useless to a group of nomads in the desert, because they are incapable of using the technology. However, it's always better to have the basics and building blocks around just in case they can or will be needed, right?

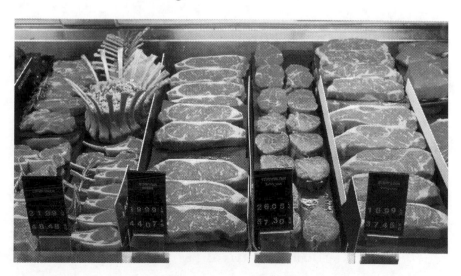

I could go into all of the complex biochemical processes, cycles, and pathways that involve the utilization of amino acids and proteins. However, since these topics have already been adequately covered in many other nutrition books, textbooks, and reference materials, I'd just like to cover some of the basics and essentials here and provide you with a simple set of take-home points for proteins and amino acids in the context of dieting and weight-management strategies. Many of these recommendations and opinions are similar to those provided when discussing the dietary intake of both sugars and fats. However, quite a few of them are unique.

The most important things we will discuss here regarding amino acids and proteins are the following topics:

- the twenty amino acids
- the essential amino acids
- the best sources of essential amino acids
- the most important processes completed by proteins and amino acids
- the benefits of amino acid supplementation
- the role of amino acids and enzymes as messengers
- the role of amino acids in neurotransmission between cells and tissues
- current studies regarding amino acids in health

- muscle recovery and muscle loss prevention
- proteins, amino acids, and weight management
- genetically modified proteins, amino acids, and bases.

The human body requires twenty different amino acids to carry out its needed biochemical processes and functions on a daily basis. According to the National Research Council, amino acids are required for the synthesis of body protein and other important nitrogen-containing compounds, such as creatinine, peptide hormones, and some neurotransmitters. And although daily nutritional allowances are expressed as protein, the biological requirement is for amino acids. So, it's really all about these twenty amino acids.

Of these twenty amino acids required by the human body, nine of them are considered to be dietarily essential because, unlike the other eleven amino acids, they cannot be made by the human body. The human body has the ability to break down proteins and amino acids and use the breakdown products to manufacture eleven of the amino acids (of the twenty) the body requires. However, at the moment, the human body is incapable of manufacturing the remaining nine essential amino acids: valine, leucine, isoleucine, lysine, methionine, threonine, phenylalanine, tryptophan, and histidine. These nine amino acids must be acquired daily from the foods we eat, although some other amino acids may become essential because of specific metabolic disorders.

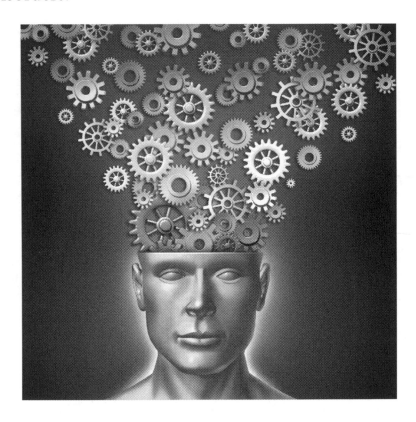

Of these nine amino acids, three are characterized as branched-chain amino acids (BCAAs): leucine, isoleucine, and valine (their first letters create the initialism LIV). These three amino acids represent a large percentage of the human body's total store and need for amino acids. Unlike most other amino acids, which are broken down within the liver, the BCAAs are mostly broken down within muscle tissues. Because of this circumstance, they are thought to play a role in energy production during exercise and, hence, during fat breakdown processes. Given this possibility, they may have the ability to reduce physical and mental fatigue and improve muscle mass, and may help to promote weight loss and tighter control of blood sugar levels (which, consequently, also promotes weight management and aids in the prevention of diabetes). Even more specifically, they may help to prevent weight gain, while also promoting and enhancing fat breakdown since the body can use these BCAAs, instead of fats, for energy. However, additional studies are needed to confirm these hypotheses. Furthermore, additional research is needed to verify if supplements for these amino acids produce the same results as consuming them normally in the diet. Finally, the branched-chain amino acids may also help to reduce liver complications and disease associated with liver failure, including hepatic encephalopathy, since they are mostly broken down within the muscle tissues, rather than within the liver.[36]

So, what are some of the common sources of branched-chain amino acids from protein in the diet (and, hence, amino acids that comprise protein)?

---

[36] Alina Petre, "BCAA Benefits: A Review of Branched-Chain Amino Acids," November 25, 2016, Healthline, https://www.healthline.com/nutrition/bcaa.

Common sources are as follows:

- red meats, lean pork, and chicken
- beans and lentils
- milk
- tofu and tempeh
- cheeses
- eggs
- pumpkinseeds
- quinoa
- nuts.[37]

Tryptophan is needed for the production of serotonin, a chemical that acts as a neurotransmitter in the body. It is also highly significant in that it is an essential regulator of mood, sleep, and behaviors.[38] Low serotonin levels are thought to have a link to depression.

The information in the following paragraphs is adapted from material published by the National Institutes of Health:

While low serotonin levels have been linked to depressed mood and sleep disturbances, several studies have shown that supplementing with tryptophan can

---

[37] Ibid.

[38] Jenkins TA, Nguyen JC, Polglaze KE, Bertrand PP. Influence of Tryptophan and Serotonin on Mood and Cognition with a Possible Role of the Gut-Brain Axis. Nutrients. 2016;8(1):56. Published 2016 Jan 20. doi:10.3390/nu8010056

reduce symptoms of depression, boost mood, and improve sleep.[39] A nineteen-day study in sixty older women found that one gram of tryptophan per day led to increased energy and improved happiness, compared to a placebo.[40]

The three branched-chain essential amino acids are widely used to alleviate fatigue, improve athletic performance, and stimulate muscle recovery after exercise.[41] In a study of sixteen resistance-trained athletes, branched-chain amino acid supplements improved performance and muscle recovery and decreased muscle soreness, compared to a placebo.[42]

---

[39] Jenkins TA, Nguyen JC, Polglaze KE, Bertrand PP. Influence of Tryptophan and Serotonin on Mood and Cognition with a Possible Role of the Gut-Brain Axis. Nutrients. 2016;8(1):56. Published 2016 Jan 20. doi:10.3390/nu8010056

Rao TS, Asha MR, Ramesh BN, Rao KS. Understanding nutrition, depression and mental illnesses. Indian J Psychiatry. 2008;50(2):77-82. doi:10.4103/0019-5545.42391

[40] Gibson EL, Vargas K, Hogan E, et al. Effects of acute treatment with a tryptophan-rich protein hydrolysate on plasma amino acids, mood and emotional functioning in older women. Psychopharmacology (Berl). 2014;231(24):4595-4610. doi:10.1007/s00213-014-3609-z

[41] Van De Wall, MS, RD, Gavin. 5 Proven Benefits of BCAAs (Branched-Chain Amino Acids). Healthline, July 11, 2018. Retrieved from https://www.healthline.com/nutrition/benefits-of-bcaa#TOC_TITLE_HDR_2

[42] Waldron M, Whelan K, Jeffries O, Burt D, Howe L, Patterson SD. The effects of acute branched-chain amino acid supplementation on recovery from a single bout of hypertrophy exercise in resistance-trained athletes. Appl Physiol Nutr Metab. 2017 Jun;42(6):630-636. doi: 10.1139/apnm-2016-0569. Epub 2017 Jan 27. PMID: 28177706.

A recent review of eight studies has shown that supplementing with branched-chain amino acids is superior to rest in promoting muscle recovery and reducing soreness after exhaustive exercise.[43] Additionally, taking four grams of leucine per day for twelve weeks increased strength performance in untrained men, showing that essential amino acids can benefit nonathletes as well.[44]

VanDusseldorp TA, Escobar KA, Johnson KE, et al. Effect of Branched-Chain Amino Acid Supplementation on Recovery Following Acute Eccentric Exercise. Nutrients. 2018;10(10):1389. Published 2018 Oct 1. doi:10.3390/nu10101389

[43] Rahimi MH, Shab-Bidar S, Mollahosseini M, Djafarian K. Branched-chain amino acid supplementation and exercise-induced muscle damage in exercise recovery: A meta-analysis of randomized clinical trials. Nutrition. 2017 Oct;42:30-36. doi: 10.1016/j.nut.2017.05.005. Epub 2017 May 18. Erratum in: Nutrition. 2017 Dec 22;: PMID: 28870476.

VanDusseldorp TA, Escobar KA, Johnson KE, et al. Effect of Branched-Chain Amino Acid Supplementation on Recovery Following Acute Eccentric Exercise. Nutrients. 2018;10(10):1389. Published 2018 Oct 1. doi:10.3390/nu10101389

[44] National Institutes of Health (NIH). Dietary Supplements for Exercise and Athletic Performance. Fact Sheet for Health Professionals. Updated on October 17, 2019. Retrieved from https://ods.od.nih.gov/factsheets/ExerciseAndAthleticPerformance-HealthProfessional/

Mero A. Leucine supplementation and intensive training. Sports Med. 1999 Jun;27(6):347-58. doi: 10.2165/00007256-199927060-00001. PMID: 10418071.

Mobley CB, Haun CT, Roberson PA, et al. Effects of Whey, Soy or Leucine Supplementation with 12 Weeks of Resistance Training on Strength, Body Composition, and Skeletal Muscle and Adipose Tissue Histological Attributes in College-Aged Males. Nutrients. 2017;9(9):972. Published 2017 Sep 4. doi:10.3390/nu9090972

Muscle loss is a commonly seen side effect of extended illnesses and prolonged bed rest, especially in adults over the age of fifty-five.[45]

The essential amino acids have also been found to prevent muscle breakdown and preserve lean body mass.[46]

A ten-day study in twenty-two older adults on bed rest showed that those who received fifteen grams of mixed essential amino acids maintained muscle protein synthesis, while the process decreased by 30 percent in the placebo group.[47]

Essential amino acid supplements have also been found to be effective in preserving lean body mass in elderly people and athletes.[48]

---

[45] Parry SM, Puthucheary ZA. The impact of extended bed rest on the musculoskeletal system in the critical care environment. Extrem Physiol Med. 2015;4:16. Published 2015 Oct 9. doi:10.1186/s13728-015-0036-7

English KL, Paddon-Jones D. Protecting muscle mass and function in older adults during bed rest. Curr Opin Clin Nutr Metab Care. 2010;13(1):34-39. doi:10.1097/MCO.0b013e328333aa66

[46] Fujita S, Volpi E. Amino acids and muscle loss with aging. J Nutr. 2006;136(1 Suppl):277S-80S. doi:10.1093/jn/136.1.277S

Børsheim E, Bui QU, Tissier S, Kobayashi H, Ferrando AA, Wolfe RR. Effect of amino acid supplementation on muscle mass, strength and physical function in elderly. Clin Nutr. 2008;27(2):189-195. doi:10.1016/j.clnu.2008.01.001

[47] Galvan E, Arentson-Lantz E, Lamon S, Paddon-Jones D. Protecting Skeletal Muscle with Protein and Amino Acid during Periods of Disuse. Nutrients. 2016;8(7):404. Published 2016 Jul 1. doi:10.3390/nu8070404

[48] Fujita S, Volpi E. Amino acids and muscle loss with aging. J Nutr. 2006;136(1 Suppl):277S-80S. doi:10.1093/jn/136.1.277S

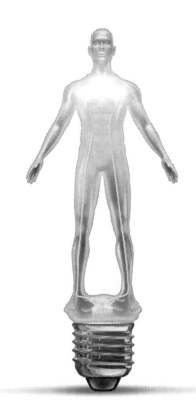

The essential amino acids may promote weight loss and may have a fat-burning effect. For instance, some human and animal studies have illustrated the ability of branched-chain essential amino acids to stimulate fat loss.[49] A two-month study in thirty-six

Dillon EL, Sheffield-Moore M, Paddon-Jones D, Gilkison C, Sanford AP, Casperson SL, Jiang J, Chinkes DL, Urban RJ. Amino acid supplementation increases lean body mass, basal muscle protein synthesis, and insulin-like growth factor-I expression in older women. J Clin Endocrinol Metab. 2009 May;94(5):1630-7. doi: 10.1210/jc.2008-1564. Epub 2009 Feb 10. PMID: 19208731; PMCID: PMC2684480.

[49] Simonson M, Boirie Y, Guillet C. Protein, amino acids and obesity treatment. Rev Endocr Metab Disord. 2020;21(3):341-353. doi:10.1007/

strength-trained men found that supplementing their diets with fourteen grams of branched-chain amino acids per day significantly decreased body fat percentages, as compared to whey protein or a sports drink.[50] A rodent study showed that a diet composed of 4 percent supplemental leucine reduced both body

s11154-020-09574-5

Novin ZS, Ghavamzadeh S, Mehdizadeh A. The Weight Loss Effects of Branched Chain Amino Acids and Vitamin B6: A Randomized Controlled Trial on Obese and Overweight Women. Int J Vitam Nutr Res. 2018 Feb;88(1-2):80-89. doi: 10.1024/0300-9831/a000511. Epub 2019 Mar 6. PMID: 30841823.

Bifari F, Ruocco C, Decimo I, Fumagalli G, Valerio A, Nisoli E. Amino acid supplements and metabolic health: a potential interplay between intestinal microbiota and systems control. Genes Nutr. 2017;12:27. Published 2017 Oct 4. doi:10.1186/s12263-017-0582-2

Valerio A, D'Antona G, Nisoli E. Branched-chain amino acids, mitochondrial biogenesis, and healthspan: an evolutionary perspective. Aging (Albany NY). 2011;3(5):464-478. doi:10.18632/aging.100322

Holeček M. Branched-chain amino acids in health and disease: metabolism, alterations in blood plasma, and as supplements. Nutr Metab (Lond). 2018;15:33. Published 2018 May 3. doi:10.1186/s12986-018-0271-1

Qin LQ, Xun P, Bujnowski D, et al. Higher branched-chain amino acid intake is associated with a lower prevalence of being overweight or obese in middle-aged East Asian and Western adults. J Nutr. 2011;141(2):249-254. doi:10.3945/jn.110.128520

[50] National Institutes of Health (NIH). Dietary Supplements for Exercise and Athletic Performance. Fact Sheet for Health Professionals. Updated on October 17, 2019. Retrieved from https://ods.od.nih.gov/factsheets/ExerciseAndAthleticPerformance-HealthProfessional/

VanDusseldorp TA, Escobar KA, Johnson KE, et al. Effect of Branched-Chain Amino Acid Supplementation on Recovery Following Acute Eccentric Exercise. Nutrients. 2018;10(10):1389. Published 2018 Oct 1. doi:10.3390/nu10101389

weight and body fat percentages.[51] However, other clinical trials and studies investigating the potential links between the branched-chain amino acids, weight loss, and body fat have been inconsistent in their findings. Therefore, additional studies are needed to determine if these amino acids can consistently promote weight loss across various populations.[52]

Mero A. Leucine supplementation and intensive training. Sports Med. 1999 Jun;27(6):347-58. doi: 10.2165/00007256-199927060-00001. PMID: 10418071.

Helms ER, Aragon AA, Fitschen PJ. Evidence-based recommendations for natural bodybuilding contest preparation: nutrition and supplementation. J Int Soc Sports Nutr. 2014;11:20. Published 2014 May 12. doi:10.1186/1550-2783-11-20

51   Ribeiro RV, Solon-Biet SM, Pulpitel T, et al. Of Older Mice and Men: Branched-Chain Amino Acids and Body Composition. Nutrients. 2019;11(8):1882. Published 2019 Aug 13. doi:10.3390/nu11081882

Pedroso JA, Zampieri TT, Donato J Jr. Reviewing the Effects of L-Leucine Supplementation in the Regulation of Food Intake, Energy Balance, and Glucose Homeostasis. Nutrients. 2015;7(5):3914-3937. Published 2015 May 22. doi:10.3390/nu7053914

Cummings NE, Williams EM, Kasza I, et al. Restoration of metabolic health by decreased consumption of branched-chain amino acids. J Physiol. 2018;596(4):623-645. doi:10.1113/JP275075

Hu C, Li F, Duan Y, Yin Y, Kong X. Dietary Supplementation With Leucine or in Combination With Arginine Decreases Body Fat Weight and Alters Gut Microbiota Composition in Finishing Pigs. Front Microbiol. 2019;10:1767. Published 2019 Aug 13. doi:10.3389/fmicb.2019.01767

52   Holeček M. Branched-chain amino acids in health and disease: metabolism, alterations in blood plasma, and as supplements. Nutr Metab (Lond). 2018;15:33. Published 2018 May 3. doi:10.1186/s12986-018-0271-1

VanDusseldorp TA, Escobar KA, Johnson KE, et al. Effect of Branched-Chain Amino Acid Supplementation on Recovery Following Acute Eccentric Exercise. Nutrients. 2018;10(10):1389. Published 2018 Oct 1. doi:10.3390/nu10101389

In general, I would recommend a combination of these foods in order to obtain the necessary quantities of branched-chain (and other) amino acids on a daily basis. However, because of some of the information provided in the chapter on fats (specifically, the parts about omega fatty acids) and because of research on sources of inflammation (which tends to promote the maintenance of additional weight), I would recommend a preference for some sources of amino acids (and, hence, proteins) over others.

In general, I would recommend that your sources of daily protein be principally composed of the following:

- vegetables, even though they also provide fiber and other nutrients
- fish, poultry, and lean red meats
- pumpkinseeds
- nuts
- quinoa.

As far as I'm concerned, the jury is still out on tofu and tempeh (unless they have been a stable, consistent part of a lifestyle and weight-management strategy that you're satisfied with). According to Ecowatch, "Tempeh is high in soy protein, which can promote satiety, reduce hunger and increase weight loss. Tempeh is traditionally made from soybeans, which contain natural plant compounds called isoflavones. Soy isoflavones have been associated with reduced cholesterol levels."[53] They are also known to contain probiotics, which may also help to promote weight loss and healthy GI tract flora.

However, other data suggests that soy/tofu products also promote inflammatory processes within the body. So the key here is balance. I would not recommend that the vast majority of your diet come from soy sources.[54]

Vegetables are important because they generally contain lower percentages of fat and because they contain pigments, isoflavones, and phytonutrients that are thought to promote the prevention of cancer and to enhance weight management. I would also highly recommend a diet that includes fresh fish that is baked or broiled (not fried) several times each week. However, in general, I would recommend limiting your daily and weekly intake of red meat (unless it specifically works for you, i.e., it appears to help you promote weight management). But I do recommend that some lean red meat be consumed during the week or else in small amounts on a daily basis. Additionally, I recommend the daily intake

---

[53] "6 Reasons Tempeh Should Be Part of a Healthy Diet," May 22, 2017, Ecowatch, https://www.ecowatch.com/tempeh-healthy-diet-2418024546.html.

[54] "6 Reasons Tempeh Should Be Part of a Healthy Diet," Ecowatch, May 22, 2017, https://www.ecowatch.com/tempeh-healthy-diet-2418024546.html.

of primarily white meat chicken, preferably natural, raised without hormones or antibiotics. Furthermore, I would strongly recommend the consumption of beans, lentils, pumpkinseeds, quinoa, and nuts.

I recommend these because I strongly believe that the closer your diet is to the most natural sources of nutrients, the better (and, hence, cleaner) it is, and the more strongly it will promote healthy weight management. I believe that good diets contain nutrients and biochemicals that are healthy and weight-management-friendly and help to prevent inflammatory responses.

However, it has been suggested that some of the common protein sources are associated with inflammatory responses and processes, which may help to promote both weight gain and fat and water retention.

According to the Lung Health Institute, the following twenty-one foods tend to promote inflammatory responses and mucus production:

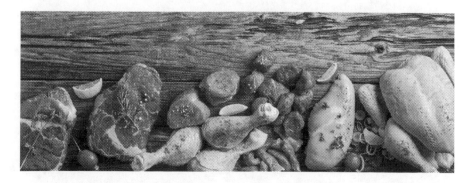

- red meats
- milk
- cheeses
- yogurt
- ice cream
- butter
- eggs
- bread
- pasta
- cereal
- bananas
- cabbage
- potatoes
- corn, corn syrup, and other corn products
- soy products
- sweet desserts
- candy
- coffee
- tea
- soda
- alcoholic beverages.[55]

Furthermore, According to the Lung Health Institute, the following twenty-one foods tend to deter and reduce inflammatory responses and mucus production:

---

[55] Lung Health, "21 Foods that Trigger Mucus Production (and 21 Foods that Reduce It)," December 26, 2017, Lung Institute, https://lunginstitute. com/blog/21-foods-trigger-mucus-production-21-foods-reduce/.2017.

- salmon
- tuna
- sardines
- flounder
- pumpkin and pumpkinseeds
- grapefruit
- pineapple
- watercress
- celery
- pickles
- onions
- garlic
- honey, agar, and agave nectars
- ginger
- lemon
- cayenne pepper
- chamomile
- olive oil
- broth
- decaf tea
- water.[56]

Of course, the number one method of reducing inflammation is to consistently intake clean water!

So, what's left to cover in this chapter? (1) The most important processes completed by proteins and amino

---

[56] Ibid.

acids, (2) the benefits of amino acid supplementation, (3) the role of amino acids as messengers, (4) the role of amino acids in neurotransmission between cells and tissues, (5) current studies regarding amino acids in health, (6) muscle recovery and muscle loss prevention, (7) proteins, amino acids, and weight management, and (8) genetically modified proteins, amino acids, and bases.

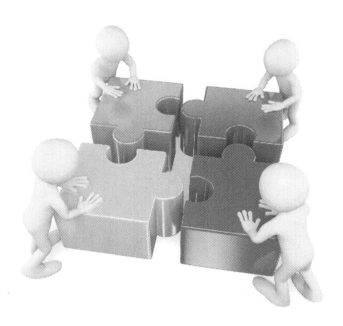

The most important processes completed by proteins and amino acids are communication and the building of bodily structures, tissues, and organs. Proteins are needed to help construct tissues and organs within the entire body and to replace and/or repair them regularly.

In a sense, proteins are like bricks. However, in addition, they are present in membranes as gatekeepers and security guards. Indeed, they help to control which substances are allowed into cells and tissues and which substances are barred from entry. So, they help to perform regulatory and security functions by controlling the entry and exit of things into and out of cells and tissues, including ions (such as Na+, Ca+, and Cl−) and other nutrients (such as vitamins and minerals).

Perhaps the most important roles that proteins and amino acids play is as messengers, communicators, and activators. Proteins known as enzymes allow for communication between different cells, tissues, organs, and organ systems. In this way, they function as messengers to convey information from one part of the body to other parts (similar to the way hormones and neurotransmitters do). These messengers have the effect of regulating the production of other enzymes and proteins, hormones, neurotransmitters (which may contain amino acids and/or proteins), ions, vitamins and minerals, and body fluids (such as water, blood, and lymph). Furthermore, they also help to regulate biochemical responses and immune responses.

In addition, one of the most important roles played by proteins, amino acids, and enzymes is that of gene activation. This brings up a really important point, one that is conveyed by Dr. Bruce Lipton in the book *The Biology of Belief.* DNA and genes are only as important as their ability to become activated by a stimulus (i.e., a cause). If genes aren't able or capable of receiving an environmental signal, then they will never be activated. Then they will remain dormant, unable to fulfill their potential, duty, or functions. Therefore, the presence and availability of enzymes (and, hence, proteins) is absolutely vital for your genes to become activated in order to perform the functions they were designed to perform. In other words, no stimulus, no response; no cause, no effect; no action, no reaction. Proteins, enzymes, and amino acids are also potent activators of biochemical reactions. They help to regulate hundreds, and perhaps thousands, of biochemical reactions, processes, and cycles that are vital to a healthy metabolism and the sustenance of a purposeful life. Without them, death would certainly result. They are regulators in the biochemistry of the human body.

Proteins, amino acids, and enzymes play a vital role in DNA. They assist in the ability of the human species to pass genes from one generation to the next, thereby helping to ensure the perpetuation and success of the human species.

Proteins and amino acids also help to form neurotransmitters—the messengers that the central nervous system (brain and spinal cord) and the peripheral nervous system (all nervous tissues residing outside the brain and spinal cord) use for communication with other nervous tissues and with other parts of the body. Without them, life would not be possible. As mentioned earlier, certain amino acids (i.e., the branched-chain amino acids: valine, leucine, and isoleucine) also play important roles in maintaining muscle tissues and preventing the breakdown of muscle tissues when additional energy is needed, thereby promoting the breakdown of fat (glycogen) instead. Finally, just as it is important to limit sugars and fats, it's important to avoid the consumption of highly modified, processed, and/or genetically engineered proteins and amino acids so that the body won't see them as foreign and then initiate an immune response leading to autoimmune disease.

This brings up another important point: Should you supplement your diet with amino acids, proteins, and/or enzymes? In general, I do recommend that you supplement your diet with the necessary amino acids if you have the habit of eating improperly (i.e., consuming meals that don't contain everything that your body needs for the day). However, if you have a proven track record (i.e., you've been able to consume all [or a high percentage] of your daily nutrient and substance requirements every day for at least sixty to ninety days), then a supplement may not be necessary. It makes a lot of sense to take a supplement on days when you know that you are going to cheat, or when you go on vacation, or when you are engaged in other activities that lead to inconsistencies in your daily consumption habits. Furthermore, it's important to consume enough water so that your body can rid itself of quantities of consumption that cannot be stored and are beyond what is required by the body for that day.

Perhaps the important concept to keep in mind here is the extinction principle, which states that when you provide your body with something on a regular basis, your body is less likely (and, therefore, less prepared) to make the substance itself (like when you give your kid an allowance without his or her having to do anything to earn it). This is the case with proteins, enzymes, neurotransmitters, biochemical messengers, and hormones. If you give them to the body on a regular basis, then you take away the stimulus (which, in this case, is the lack of something) that leads to its production. The phrase "full dogs don't hunt" expresses this principle.

So, keep this in mind when you make the choice to supplement your diet with substances and chemicals that the body normally produces. It you do the work for the body, then it will learn that it doesn't need to do the work itself (this is called conditioning). This is at the heart of gene activation theories and Dr. Bruce Lipton's *The Biology of Belief*. Moreover, if the stimulus (i.e., the need/lack) disappears, then so will the response (fulfillment of the need). Therefore, I recommend that even if you choose to take supplements, you take vacation days or weeks here and there just to remind your body that it still needs to make certain things such as amino acids, neurotransmitters, and hormones—if it is able to.

In direct contrast, for example, if you have a loss of thyroid function and you have to supplement your metabolism with thyroxine, then taking a break from thyroxine won't work because your body isn't able to make it. However, if you take a sleep aid either occasionally or regularly, just keep in mind that your body will stop making the chemicals and substances needed to induce and maintain sleep if you give such chemicals and substances to your body regularly. Because of this, it's not wise to take prescription sleep aids on a regular basis in my opinion. You should at least take a break from both stimulants (such as coffee) and relaxants (such as sleep aids) on weekends and during vacations. I cover this topic in my first book, *Sweet Potato Pie for the Spirit, Soul, and Psyche*— which contains a short, concise chapter on sleep, sleep disorders, sleep mechanics and biochemistry, and sleep solutions.

At any rate, the extinction principle is a concept that governs the entire human body and all its functions. If you do the work for the metabolism—that is, if you give your body what it normally makes on its own—then your body will gradually learn to stop making it since there is no longer a need for it to do so. In other words, don't blame your body from learning from your habits and rituals.

In terms of diet, nutrition, and lifestyle principles for proteins and amino acids, the most important concepts in terms of weight management are the following:

- avoiding nonnatural proteins, amino acids, and enzymes that may be present in genetically modified food products;
- leaning toward the consumption of vegetables, fish, poultry, pumpkinseeds, nuts, and quinoa as primary protein sources;
- avoiding protein sources that tend to lead to inflammatory states and process, which in turn lead to mucus production and the maintenance of water;

- using amino acid, protein, and enzyme supplements wisely, such that the body is encouraged to keep making what it needs— which, in and of itself, helps to burn calories and consume energy.

Remember that your body needs the necessarily stimuli to lose weight and maintain preferred levels of metabolic activity. Therefore, use both diet (e.g., the consumption of branched-chain amino acids) and activity (physical activity, exercise, aerobics, and sports) to stimulate the desired genes to promote fat-burning and other metabolic activities.

Keep in mind that your body will use the biochemical pathways associated with gluconeogenesis to convert amino acids and proteins into energy (i.e., glucose, and hence, ATP). Essentially, if you give the body too much protein, then it will stop relying on burning fat (i.e., glycogen) for energy. So, keep your protein calories in check so that your body will use fat (i.e., glycogen) for fuel rather than dietary protein, especially late in the daytime. Consume most of your fat, carbohydrate, and protein calories during the earlier parts of the day, and gradually switch to more fruits, vegetables, and fiber-containing foods as the day progresses.

CHAPTER 6

Drinks and Beverages

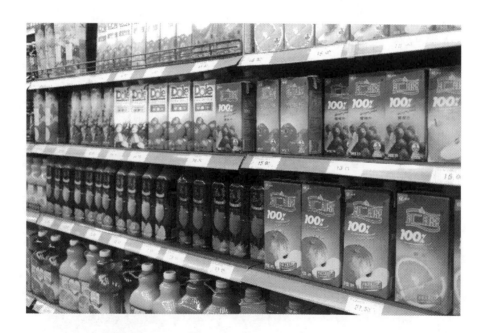

Drinks and beverages are definitely worthy of our attention. There's certainly a reason why I started *The Nutrient Diet* with a chapter about water. As I've said before, fluids are the fountains of life on this planet. And since the human body consists of two-thirds fluids, we definitely need to pay attention to the fluids that we take in and our habits associated with them. Since some specific fluids, such as water, milk, and alcohol, are covered specifically in other chapters, they will not be covered here. Consequently, this chapter will be very succinct and to the point. Generally speaking, it will present an approach to fluid intake that maximizes weight loss, weight management, and weight control while keeping the underlying foundations of health in mind. Obviously, good hydration begins with good water, which we previously covered. However, few of us consume water as the sole beverage choice.

To the contrary, most of us also consume the following (although our consumption amounts, patterns, habits, and rituals may vary vastly) beverages each year: (1) coffee, (2) tea, (3) fruit juice, (4) milk and cream, (5) soda, and (6) alcohol. As you can see in the table of contents, there is an entire chapter devoted to each water, milk/cream, and alcohol, so these beverages will only be covered in a general sense within this chapter. However, coffee, tea, fruit juice, and soda will be both generally and specifically covered in this chapter. We'll begin with soda and move backward from there.

Soft drinks (sodas, soda pops, etc.) are a staple of most American diets. As most of us are aware, they tend to be laden with either large amounts of sugar or sugar substitutes. They aren't generally healthy or advisable as a staple of any dietary or lifestyle approach. Most of us are aware of the fact that many soft drink options are saturated with sugars, but what about the diet soft drinks? That's where the discussion is most important these days. And that's easy to cover here since it's part of an important concept discussed in *The Nutrient Diet*: the more processed, chemically modified, or genetically enhanced something is, the worse it is for your metabolism and your body's ability to control fat content and stave off inflammation.

Therefore, generally speaking, I recommend that you stay away from diet soft drinks as a central (i.e., regular, ritualistic, habitual) part of your consumption habits because they tend to contain highly artificial sugar and sugar substitutes. I would recommend the consumption of smarter beverage choices. Juices are a good bet as long as they don't contain high-fructose corn syrup.

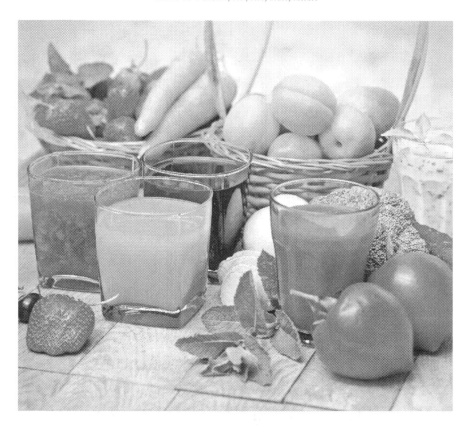

You'll have to check the labels of juices to make sure they don't contain artificial sugars or high-fructose corn syrup. Generally, if you do choose to have juices on a regular basis, I suggest that you dilute them with water. A dilution of 20 percent to 30 percent water is generally a good rule. If you do this daily, and if you consume a glass of juice three times per day on average, then you can easily eliminate two hundred to three hundred calories per day from your diet. You'll gradually get used to the lessened sweetness and the taste of the juices over time.

As suggested in the first chapter, it's always a good idea to consume a glass or two of water prior to and after having fruit juice or a meal. This will dilute your daily intake of salt and sugar and will help to keep you kidneys and renal tubules clean and healthy. Furthermore, as cited in chapter 1, the consistent consumption of water daily helps promote the breakdown of stored glycogen (i.e., adipose tissue—fat). Regardless of what beverage you consume (even if it's alcohol), it's always a good idea to have a cup or a glass of water beforehand and afterward. If you drink alcohol, diluting it by drinking water before and after helps to prevent drinking and driving and allows you to be able to leave a destination when you need or want to (or sooner than you might otherwise be able to).

I often hear from my clients that they can't remember to drink water throughout the day. Depending on your level of activity, focus, and/or concentration during the day, you may have a valid excuse for forgetting to drink water. In any event, here's an *easy* solution: throughout the day, as you work, listen to relaxation or subliminal audio tracks that mimic the sound of ocean waves, mountain streams, or running water currents. That's what I do. Those sounds, while tending to blend into the background and induce calm and collectiveness throughout my day, also continuously remind to me to get another glass of water. It's an *easy* mental connection and a viable solution to counter the excuse that you can't remember to drink water. Another strategy is to have Post-it Notes and images in your workspace that remind you to drink water.

In reference to fruit juice, keep in mind that many people have allergies to common foodstuffs and to plants, weeds, grasses, and trees. Keep in mind that high levels of consumption of certain fruit juices could be contributing to an inflammatory state. If you find certain juices to be highly acidic, then either stay away from them, significantly dilute them, or drink lots of water in between drinking them. In addition, as will be covered in the chapter on alcoholic beverages, if you desire a rum and Coke, then have a rum and Coke instead of a rum and Diet Coke. Just drink more water between drinks. It's better to wash the more natural sugars away with water than to intake the unnatural sugars.

CHAPTER 7

Alcohol and Other Relaxants

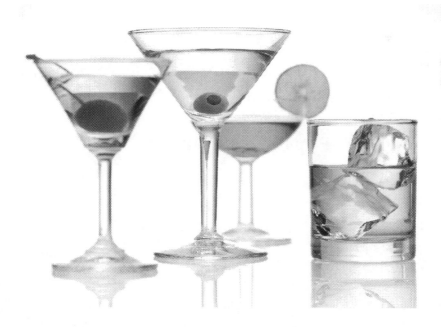

The Following are thirty-one rules and resources for responsible alcohol consumption &/or hangover prevention. It should be noted that many of the concepts that prevent hangovers are also consistent with more responsible drinking behaviors and with cognitive control of calories associated with alcohol consumption. Generally speaking, responsible drinking and responsible eating go hand in hand; they compliment one another. Finally, this chapter is included because it includes important information about alcohol, and alcohol is a consistent part of the diet of most drinking-age Americans (and Europeans, for that matter).

1. Drink in moderation or not at all.

2. Avoid drinks with congeners, the toxic by-products of alcohol production.

3. Thinking of having a drink the morning after? Don't! Just don't.

4. Drink plenty of water.

5. Get enough sleep.

6. Eat a hearty, healthy breakfast containing fiber.

7. Take supplements that might help, such as prickly pear.

8. All the bubbles in sparkling wine are carbon dioxide. The CO_2 competes with oxygen in our bloodstream, says one researcher, who studies the effects of alcohol on the body. According to a Princeton University explainer of alcohol

absorption, carbon dioxide "increases the pressure in your stomach, forcing alcohol out through the lining of your stomach into the bloodstream. That can speed up the rate of alcohol absorption—albeit temporarily. So if you want to stay steady on your feet, sip that bubbly slowly. And if you want to prevent a hangover, swap your next glass of bubbly for water. Alternating between alcoholic beverages and H_2O can help prevent the dehydration that accompanies a night of drinking."[57]

9. Remember, your actual cocktail may be equal to two, three, four, or *more* drinks (based on the personality and habits of the bartender [the bartender being the individual who prepared your drink, licensed bartender or not])!

10. Take vitamins and minerals with your breakfast, not by themselves.

   "High levels of alcohol in the brain have fairly recently been shown to cause neuro-inflammation, basically, inflammation in the brain." This is why taking aspirin or other anti-inflammatory medicines, such as ibuprofen, can help us feel better.[58]

---

57   *The Wine Spectator*, November 20, 2017.
58   Allison Aubrey, "Want to Avoid a Hangover? Science Has Got You Covered," NPR, December 31, 2015, http://

Now, alcohol isn't the only headache-producing culprit in our drinking glasses. Many alcoholic beverages, such as wine and beer, contain toxic by-products of fermentation such as aldehydes. Tabakoff says that if you drink too much, you can feel the effects. "If these compounds accumulate in the body," explains Tabakoff, "they can release your stress hormones, like epinephrine and norepinephrine, and as such can alter function in a stress like way"—paving the way for a hangover. Tabakoff says distilled spirits contain fewer of these toxic compounds than other types of booze, which explains why some people report feeling fewer hangover effects if they stick with vodka or gin.[59]

Adding liquid calories to your cocktails—say, Coke, ginger ale, or sugary punch as a mixer—is a good way to slow absorption too. In fact, a study from 2013 determined that a diet soda and rum will make you drunker than rum mixed with sugary Coke.[60]

Cecile Marczinski, a cognitive psychologist who authored that study, found that the average breath

www.npr.org/sections/thesalt/2015/12/31/461594898/want-to-avoid-a-hangover-science-has-got-you-covered.

[59] Ibid.

[60] Ibid.

alcohol concentration was 0.091 (at its peak) when subjects drank alcohol mixed with a diet drink. By comparison, BrAC [Breath Alcohol Concentration] was 0.077 when the same subjects consumed the same amount of alcohol but with a sugary soda. "I was a little surprised by the findings, since the 18 percent increase in [BrAC] was a fairly large difference," Marczinski reported. She says the difference would not likely have been as large if the subjects—who were all college age— had not been drinking on empty stomachs.[61]

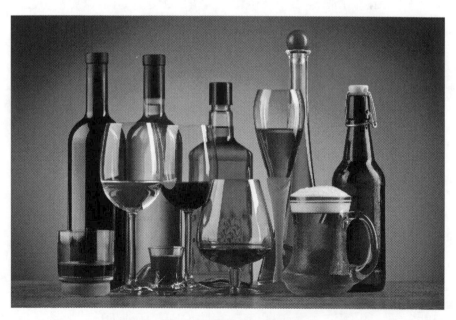

11. One drink per hour is a rule of thumb, but that can vary depending on height or body size. Bigger people tend to be able to handle a little

---

61   NPR, January 31, 2013.

more alcohol, and smaller people tend to be able to handle a little less. And remember, Tabakoff says that a single drink is more (i.e., more alcohol) than you might think.[62]

12. According to Wayne Jones, of the Swedish National Laboratory of Forensic Medicine, the biochemistry of alcohol metabolism is complicated. Jones's theory is that the liver, in processing alcohol, first addresses ethanol, which is the alcohol proper, and then moves on to methanol, a secondary ingredient of many wines and spirits. Because methanol breaks down into formic acid, which is highly toxic, it is during this second stage [i.e, the breakdown of methanol] that the hangover is most crushing. If at that point you pour in more alcohol, your body will switch back to ethanol processing. This will not eliminate the hangover—the methanol (indeed, more of it now) is still waiting for you round the bend—but it does delay the worst symptoms. It may also mitigate them somewhat. On the other hand, you are drunk again, which may create difficulty with regard to going to work.[63]

---

[62] Aubrey, "Want to Avoid a Hangover?"
[63] J. Acocella, "A Few Too Many: Is There Hope for the Hung Over?," *New Yorker*, May 26, 2008, http://www.newyorker.com/magazine/2008/05/26/a-few-too-many; *Gawker*, May 19, 2008.

13. As for the nonalcoholic means of combatting hangover, these fall into three categories: before or while drinking, before bed, and the next morning. Many people advise you to eat a heavy meal, with lots of protein and fats, before or while drinking. If you can't do that, at least drink a glass of milk. In Africa, the same purpose is served by eating peanut butter. The other most frequent before-and-during recommendation is water, lots of it. Proponents of this strategy tell you to ask for a glass of water with every drink you order and to then make yourself chugalug the water before drinking the drink.[64]

14. When you get home from a night of alcohol consumption, is there anything you can do before going to bed (to prevent a hangover)? Those still able to consider such a question are advised, again, to consume buckets of water and also to take some Vitamin C. Koreans drink a bowl of water with honey, presumably to head off the hypoglycemia.[65]

15. Elsewhere on the international front, many people in Asia and the Near East take strong tea. The Italians and the French prefer strong

---

[64] Acocella, "A Few Too Many"; *Medical News Today*, October 17, 2017.
[65] *New Yorker*, May 19, 2008.

coffee. (Italian informant: add lemon. French informant: add salt. Alcohol researchers: stay away from coffee—it's a diuretic and will make you more dehydrated.) Germans eat pickled herring; the Japanese turn to pickled plums; the Vietnamese drink a juice from the wax gourd. Moroccans say to chew cuminseeds; Andeans, coca leaves. Russians swear by pickle brine. An ex-Soviet ballet dancer told me, "Pickle juice or a shot of vodka or pickle juice with a shot of vodka." Many folk cures for hangovers are soups: menudo in Mexico, *mondongo* in Puerto Rico, *işkembe çorbasi* in Turkey, *patsa* in Greece, *khashi* in Georgia. The fact that all these dishes involve tripe may mean something. Hungarians favor a concoction of cabbage and smoked meats, sometimes forthrightly called "hangover soup." The Russians' morning-after soup, *solyanka*, is, of course, made with pickle juice.[66]

16. Many hangover cures—the soups, the greasy breakfast—are comfort foods, and that, apart from any sworn-by ingredients, may be their chief therapeutic property. But some other remedies sound as though they were devised by the witches in *Macbeth*.[67]

---

[66] *New Yorker*, October 20, 2010; *New Yorker*, May 19, 2008.
[67] *New Yorker*, May 19, 2008.

17. The most widely used over-the-counter (OTC) remedy is no doubt aspirin. Advil, or ibuprofen, and Alka-Seltzer—there is a special formula for hangovers, namely, Alka-Seltzer Wake-Up Call—are probably close runners-up. (Tylenol, or acetaminophen, should not be used because alcohol increases its toxicity to the liver.) Also commonly recommended are vitamin C and B-complex vitamins. But those are almost home remedies. In recent years, pharmaceutical companies have come up with more specialized formulas: Chaser, NoHang, BoozEase, PartySmart, Sob'r-K Hangover Stopper, Hangover Prevention Formula, and so on. In some of these, such as Sob'r-K and Chaser, the primary ingredient is carbon, which, according to the manufacturers, soaks up toxins. Others are herbal compounds, featuring such ingredients as ginseng, milk thistle, borage, and extracts of prickly pear, artichoke, and guava leaf. These and other OTC remedies aim to boost biochemicals that help the body deal with toxins. A few remedies have scientific backing. Manuela Neuman, in lab tests, found that milk thistle extract, which is an ingredient in NoHang and Hangover Helper, does protect cells from damage by alcohol. A research team headed by Jeffrey Wiese, of Tulane University, tested extract of prickly pear, the key ingredient

in Hangover Prevention Formula, on human subjects and found significant improvement with the nausea, dry mouth, and food aversion but not with other, more common symptoms such as headache.[68]

18. Most cures for hangover—indeed, most statements about hangover—have not been tested. Jeffrey Wiese and his colleagues, in a 2000 article in *Annals of Internal Medicine*, reported that in the preceding thirty-five years, more than forty-seven hundred articles on alcohol intoxication had been published, but only one hundred eight of these dealt with hangover. There may be more information on hangover cures in college newspapers—a rich source—than in the scientific literature. And the research that has been published is often weak. A team of scientists attempting to review the literature on hangover cures were able to assemble only fifteen articles, and then they had to throw out all but eight on methodological grounds. There have been more studies in recent years, but historically this is not a subject that has captured scientists' hearts.[69]

---

[68]   GoodRx, November 21, 2018; CNN, December 31, 2010; *New Yorker*, May 19, 2008.

[69]   *New Yorker*, May 19, 2008; the *New York Times*, December 27, 2000; *Annals of Internal Medicine* (2000); WebMD, June 5, 2000; J. Howland, NCBI/NIH, 2008; *Science* (January 9, 2004).

19. A refreshing can of ginger ale or a Sprite.

20. The best alcohol absorber: *food!*

21. The following is according to *Medical News Today*:

- The previously elusive "hangover cure" remains elusive.
- Eating food before a drinking session is a must.
- Pacing yourself with a glass of water can help.
- Avoid taking Tylenol on a hangover.
- Sports drinks might help reduce some symptoms.
- A preemptive ibuprofen can help minimize symptoms.
- Prehydration and rehydration are *key!*[70]

22. The following is according to Greatist:

- Refuel at the breakfast table. Alcohol will lead to a drop in blood sugar, so boost your blood sugar back up with a glass of apple juice in the morning. Fruit juices are a good way to treat mild low blood sugar, but if the situation feels dire, then choose something with a high

---

[70] *Discover* magazine, May 30, 2018; British Columbia Drug and Poison Information Centre, 2014.

glycemic index, such as dark horse Rice Chex or a French baguette.

- Go one-for-one. It's no secret that drinking water can help deflect that pounding morning headache (pretty much the opposite of a good morning). Tissues around the brain are mostly made of water, and dehydration will shrink these tissues, creating pressure in the head. Alcohol can lead to dehydration, so make sure to continuously drink water throughout the night. Try matching each alcoholic drink with one glass of water to avoid that next-day pain.

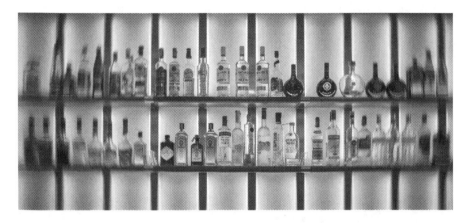

- Chow down. Just because beer has calories doesn't mean it counts as dinner. Drinking on an empty stomach will allow alcohol to absorb faster, so try getting in a good meal with lots of healthy carbs before breaking out the bottle. Some research even shows a stomach full of food may help keep blood alcohol content at a lower level.

- Keep it light. Darker drinks such as red wine or rum contain more congeners (substances produced during fermentation), which may contribute to causing hangovers. Skip the whiskey in favor of vodka or a glass of white wine!

- Stay classy. The more expensive liquors are usually distilled more times, so they contain fewer congeners—as we just learned, a cause for the shaking-one's-fist-at-the-sky action. So pass on the well liquor and take it up a notch with some top-shelf booze.

- Take a multivitamin. Drinking depletes nutrients in the body, including vitamin B_{12} and folate. Try popping in a multivitamin to replenish what's lost from a night of drinking.

- Skip the bubbles. Opt out of champagne or other alcohol that's mixed with carbonated beverages. Research shows that the bubbles may cause alcohol to be absorbed more quickly, hence that New Year's Day hangover.

- Practice your downward dog. Scientists have yet to prove that a few sun salutations will whisk away a hangover, but breathing and meditation exercises in yoga can get oxygen flowing and blood pumping to help relieve stress, usually abundant when the world feels sideways.

- Grab some potassium. When dehydrated, we lose not only water but also electrolytes. Gain 'em back by snacking on potassium-rich foods such as bananas or spinach. And if you're thinking ahead, stock up on Pedialyte—one bottle has twice the sodium and five times as much potassium as the same size bottle of Gatorade.

- Scramble eggs. Eggs contain taurine, which has been shown to reverse liver damage caused by a night of heavy boozing. Scramble them up with lots of veggies for added antioxidant power!

- Sip ginger tea. Hangovers sometimes come with a side of upset stomach, so try a warm mug of ginger tea to settle things down. Ginger has been shown to help combat nausea.

- Get some fresh air. Oxygen increases the rate at which alcohol toxins are broken down, so bundle up and get outdoors. A little exercise never hurt anyone—and it may even release some endorphins to boost that posthangover mood.

- Play designated driver. The only surefire way to avoid a hangover is to skip the booze altogether. So if waking up to a pounding headache doesn't sound fun, play designated driver for the night (even if not actually driving). At the very least, you'll have some great stories to tell.[71]

23. The following is according to Caron:

Alcohol (also known as ethanol or ethyl alcohol) is a psychoactive drug that acts as a central nervous system depressant. Alcohol interferes with communication between nerve cells and all other cells and affects various centers in the brain. Even moderate consumption of alcohol causes immediate effects, such as lowered inhibitions, increased relaxation, and dulled senses.[72]

As alcohol consumption (and blood alcohol) increases, users may experience:

- heightened emotional responses (including anger and aggression)
- lack of coordination
- poor balance
- slurred speech
- dizziness
- disturbed sleep

---

[71] Kathy Warwick, "13 Legitimate Ways to Stop a Hangover," July 24, 2015, the Greatist, https://greatist.com/health/13-legit-ways-stop-hangover.
[72] Caron Treatment Centers.

- nausea and vomiting.[73]

Alcohol affects the body in stages, causing various states of being, including:

- relaxation
- euphoria
- excitement
- confusion
- stupor.[74]

Extreme alcohol consumption can cause memory loss (blackouts), complete loss of coordination, and alcohol poisoning. In some cases, alcohol overdose can be fatal. Other short-term effects of alcohol include harm to the body's tissues:

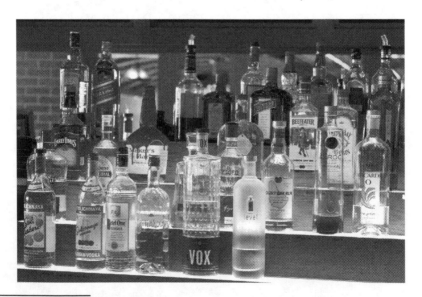

---

[73] Alcohol.org, October 23, 2019.
[74] Ibid.

- Stomach
Alcohol irritates the stomach and intestine lining and increases stomach acid secretion. This causes vomiting.

- Skin
Alcohol increases blood flow to the skin, causing users to sweat and appear flushed.

- Muscles
Alcohol and reduces blood flow to the muscles, causing muscle aches (most notably felt as the alcohol leaves the system.) This effect is often called a hangover.

The severity of the effects of alcohol is dependent on a variety of factors, including the weight, age, and sex of the individual consuming the alcohol and how much was eaten before and during consumption. Alcohol is eventually metabolized and eliminated from the system at a rate of 13 mg to 18 mg per hour.[75]

24. The following is according to the National Institutes of Health (NIH):

---

[75] National Institute on Alcohol Abuse and Alcoholism, "Alcohol's Effects on the Body," October 2004, National Institutes of Health, https://www.niaaa.nih.gov/alcohol-health/alcohols-effects-body.

Drinking too much—on a single occasion or over time—can take a serious toll on your health. Here's how alcohol can affect your body:

Brain

Alcohol interferes with the brain's communication pathways and may affect the way the brain looks and works. These disruptions can change mood and behavior, and make it harder to think clearly and move with coordination.[76]

Heart

Drinking a lot over a long time or too much on a single occasion can damage the heart, causing problems, including the following:

- cardiomyopathy—stretching and drooping of heart muscle
- arrhythmia—irregular heartbeat
- stroke
- high blood pressure.

Research also shows that drinking moderate amounts of alcohol may protect healthy adults from developing coronary heart disease.[77]

---

[76] Ibid.

[77] Ibid.

Liver

Heavy drinking takes a toll on the liver and can lead to a variety of problems and liver inflammations, including the following:

- steatosis, or fatty liver
- alcoholic hepatitis
- fibrosis
- cirrhosis.[78]

Pancreas

Alcohol causes the pancreas to produce toxic substances. This can eventually lead to pancreatitis, a dangerous inflammation and swelling of the blood vessels in the pancreas that prevents proper digestion.[79]

Cancer

Drinking too much alcohol can increase your risk of developing certain cancers, including cancers of the following:

- mouth
- esophagus
- throat

---

[78] Ibid.
[79] Ibid.

- liver
- breast.[80]

Immune System

Drinking too much can weaken your immune system, making your body a much easier target for disease. Chronic drinkers are more liable to contract diseases such as pneumonia and tuberculosis than people who do not drink too much. Drinking a lot on a single occasion slows your body's ability to ward off infections—even up to twenty-four hours after getting drunk.[81]

25. The following is according to Healthline:

One glass of alcohol a day may do little damage to your overall health. But if the habit grows or if you find yourself having a hard time stopping after just one glass, the cumulative effects can add up.[82] These effects include the following:

Damage to the Digestive System and Endocrine Glands

Drinking too much alcohol can cause abnormal activation of digestive enzymes produced by

---

[80] Ibid.

[81] Ibid.

[82] Healthline, June 9, 2017; *New York Times*, October 24, 2019.

the pancreas. Buildup of these enzymes can lead to inflammation known as pancreatitis. Pancreatitis can become a long-term condition and cause serious complications.[83]

Inflammatory Damage

The liver is an organ that helps break down and remove harmful substances from your body, including alcohol. Long-term alcohol use interferes with this process. It also increases your risk for chronic liver inflammation and liver disease. The scarring caused by this inflammation is known as cirrhosis. The formation of scar tissue destroys the liver. As the liver becomes increasingly damaged, it has a harder time removing toxic substances from your body. Liver disease is life-threatening and leads to toxins and waste buildup in your body. Women are at higher risk for developing alcoholic liver disease. Women's bodies are more likely to absorb more alcohol and need longer periods of time to process it. Women also show liver damage more quickly than men.[84]

---

[83] Ibid.
[84] Ibid.

Sugar Levels

The pancreas helps regulate your body's insulin use and response to glucose. When your pancreas and liver aren't functioning properly, you run the risk of experiencing low blood sugar, or hypoglycemia. A damaged pancreas may also prevent the body from producing enough insulin to utilize sugar. This can lead to hyperglycemia, or too much sugar in the blood. If your body can't manage and balance your blood sugar levels, you may experience greater complications and side effects related to diabetes. It's important for people with diabetes or hypoglycemia to avoid excessive amounts of alcohol.[85]

Central Nervous System

One of the easiest ways to obtain a glimpse of alcohol's impact on your body is to notice, understand and appreciate how it affects your central nervous system. Slurred speech is one of the first signs you've had too much to drink. Alcohol can reduce communication between your brain and your body. This makes coordination more difficult. You may have a hard time balancing. You should never drive after drinking.

---

[85] Ibid.

As alcohol causes more damage to your central nervous system, you may experience numbness and tingling sensations in your feet and hands. Drinking also makes it difficult for your brain to create long-term memories. It also reduces your ability to think clearly and make rational choices. Over time, frontal lobe damage can occur. This area of the brain is responsible for emotional control, short-term memory, and judgment, in addition to other vital roles. Chronic and severe alcohol abuse can also cause permanent brain damage. This can lead to Wernicke–Korsakoff syndrome, a brain disorder that affects memory.[86]

Dependency

Some people who drink heavily may develop a physical and emotional dependency on alcohol. Alcohol withdrawal can be difficult and life-threatening. One often needs professional help to break an alcohol addiction. As a result, many people seek medical detoxification to get sober. This is the safest way to ensure you break the physical addiction. Depending on the risk for withdrawal symptoms, detoxification can be managed on either an outpatient or inpatient basis. Symptoms of alcohol withdrawal include:

---

[86]   Ibid.

- anxiety
- nervousness
- nausea
- tremors
- high blood pressure
- irregular heartbeat
- heavy sweating.

Seizures, hallucinations, and delirium may occur in severe cases of withdrawal.[87]

Digestive System

The connection between alcohol consumption and your digestive system might not seem immediately clear. The side effects often only appear after there has been damage. And the more you drink, the greater the damage will become. Drinking can damage the tissues in your digestive tract and prevent your intestines from digesting food and absorbing nutrients and vitamins. As a result, malnutrition may occur. Heavy drinking can also lead to the following:

- gassiness
- bloating
- a feeling of fullness in your abdomen

---

[87] Ibid.

- diarrhea or painful stools.[88]

For people who drink heavily, ulcers or hemorrhoids (a result of dehydration and constipation) aren't uncommon. And these may cause dangerous internal bleeding. Ulcers can be fatal if not diagnosed and treated early. People who consume too much alcohol may also be at risk for cancer. People who drink frequently are more likely to develop cancer in the mouth, throat, esophagus, colon, or liver. People who regularly drink and use tobacco together have an even greater cancer risk.[89]

Circulatory System

Alcohol can affect your heart and lungs. People who are chronic drinkers of alcohol have a higher risk of heart-related issues than people who do not drink. Women who drink are more likely to develop heart disease than men who drink. Circulatory system complications include the following:

- high blood pressure
- irregular heartbeat
- difficulty pumping blood through the body

---

88 Ibid.
89 Ibid.

- stroke
- heart attack
- heart disease
- heart failure.

Difficulty absorbing vitamins and minerals from food can cause anemia. This is a condition where you have a low red blood cell count. One of the biggest symptoms of anemia is fatigue.[90]

Sexual and Reproductive Health

You may think that drinking alcohol can lower your inhibitions and help you have more fun in bed. But the reality is quite different. Men who drink too much are more likely to experience erectile dysfunction. Heavy drinking can also prevent sex hormone production and lower your libido. Women who drink too much may stop menstruating. That puts them at a greater risk for infertility. Women who drink heavily during pregnancy have a higher risk of premature delivery, miscarriage, or stillbirth. A woman who drinks alcohol while pregnant puts her unborn child at risk. Fetal alcohol syndrome disorder (FASD) is a serious concern. Other conditions include the following:

---

[90]   Ibid.

- learning difficulties
- long-term [i.e., chronic] health conditions (such as diabetes, etc.)
- increased emotional problems
- physical development abnormalities.[91]

Skeletal and Muscle Systems

Long-term alcohol use may prevent your body from keeping your bones strong. A prolonged drinking habit may cause thinner bones and increase your risk for fractures if you fall. And any fractures may heal more slowly. Drinking alcohol may also lead to muscle weakness, cramping, and eventually atrophy.[92]

26. Drinking heavily reduces your body's natural immune system. This makes it more difficult for your body to fight off invading germs and viruses. People who drink heavily over a long period of time are also more likely to develop pneumonia or tuberculosis than the general population. About 10 percent of all tuberculosis cases worldwide can be tied to alcohol consumption. Drinking alcohol also increases your risk of several types of cancer, including of the mouth, breast, and colon.[93]

---

[91]   Ibid.

[92]   Ibid.

[93]   Ibid.

27. Quit alcohol altogether.

When someone starts out drinking, he or she feels relaxed, confident, happy, sociable. The pleasurable effects of alcohol are undeniable. It makes it easy to forget about the negative effects: slowed reflexes, reduced coordination, warped thinking, poor judgment, impaired memory, impaired motor functions, and plenty more impairments.[94]

These negative effects occur every single time one drinks, even a single beer. The more one drinks, the stronger these negative effects. (Those pleasurable effects will begin to fade quickly.) Over time, the body becomes damaged from drinking—more damaged than you probably know. In fact, alcohol can cause several types of cancer.[95]

Aside from bodily harm, alcohol use has been linked to depression, anxiety, societal withdrawal, violent behavior, an increase in unprotected sex, and increased risk of motor vehicle accidents, suicide, injury, domestic violence, and even drowning. As if that's not enough, alcohol also does unbelievable damage to the body, and not

[94]   Ibid.
[95]   Ibid.

just to the brain and liver. Virtually every part of the body is affected negatively from excessive drinking.[96]

From the First Sip

When alcohol is consumed, around 33 percent of it is absorbed immediately into the blood, through the stomach lining. The remaining alcohol is absorbed more slowly into the blood, through the small intestine. Once in the bloodstream, alcohol diffuses into almost every biological tissue in the body, because cell membranes are highly permeable.[97]

When one consumes more alcohol than his or her body can handle, that person's blood alcohol level (BAL) increases. How fast a person's BAL raises, and the effects it has, vary greatly depending on a number of things, including weight, age, gender, body composition, general health, and the presence of other drugs or medications.[98]

Regardless, the presence of alcohol in the blood at all will have effects on the body. A higher BAL simply means greater risk. The recommended

---

[96]   Ibid.
[97]   Medical News Net, February 26, 2019; Quit Alcohol, October 30, 2012.
[98]   Ibid.

maximum intake of alcohol is two drinks per day for men and one drink per day for women. Consuming more than this is considered problematic drinking. Five or more drinks per day for men, four for women, is considered binge drinking.[99]

Note: Alcoholism is a disease characterized by an inability to control alcohol use, a need to consume increasingly larger amounts of alcohol, and/or a constant impulse to consume alcohol. If this sounds familiar, please seek professional treatment immediately. With the right help, you will find that alcoholism is a 100 percent curable disease.[100]

Brain

The amount of damage alcohol causes to the brain is incomprehensible. Those little moments you don't remember from the crazy night before— that's temporary amnesia. Keep it up and you might develop Wernicke–Korsakoff syndrome (WKS), a memory-impairing, vision- and speech-affecting, seizure-causing disorder. You won't

[99] Ibid.
[100] Ibid.

be able to form new memories. You'll mumble involuntarily. Your eyes will twitch constantly.[101]

Drinking releases excess GABA and dopamine, two naturally occurring neurotransmitters. GABA is responsible for calming the brain down, and dopamine is responsible for pleasure, a part of the brain's reward system. Too much of these neurotransmitters can lead to shortness of breath, high blood pressure, increased heart rate, night terrors, delusions, hallucinations, spasms, and increased levels of both aggression and depression.[102]

Drinking also releases endorphins, which are similar to neurotransmitters, except they carry natural pain-reducing chemicals instead of messages. Endorphins are normally released upon rewarding actions, such as exercise, sexual activity, and eating. Too much endorphin release can cause depression, lower sex drive, low testosterone, infertility, and extreme fatigue, among other complications.[103]

---

[101] Quit Alcohol, October 30, 2012.
[102] Ibid.
[103] Ibid.

If you or a loved one is dependent on alcohol, please, seek immediate professional help. The following websites are a good place to start:

- https://www.webmd.com/cancer/features/faq-alcohol-and-your-health
- https://en.wikipedia.org/wiki/Long-term_effects_of_alcohol
- https://www.niaaa.nih.gov/alcohol-health
- https://www.drugabuse.gov/drugs-abuse/alcohol
- https://alcoholism.about.com/od/health/Effects_of_Alcohol_Health_Effects_of_Alcohol.htm
- https://www2.potsdam.edu/hansondj/AlcoholAndHealth.html.

28.Know your limits. Know the effects of alcohol.

Many people enjoy a drink without any problems, but binge drinking or drinking heavily over longer periods of time can have very serious consequences. Alcohol misuse not only harms the individual but also damages relationships and society in general in terms of violence, crime, accidents, and drink driving.[104]

---

[104] National Institute on Alcohol Abuse and Alcoholism, January 2006.

In Northern Ireland, the number of alcohol-related deaths has more than doubled since 1994. The most recent figures show the following:

- There were two hundred seventy deaths recorded as alcohol related in 2012.
- There were more than eleven thousand five hundred alcohol-related admissions to hospitals in 2009–10.[105]

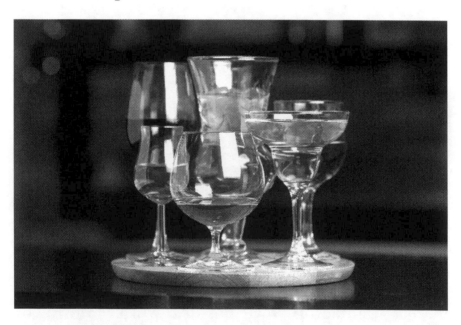

Long-Term Effects

In addition to the recognized immediate effects of drinking too much, such as nausea and vomiting, binge drinking and prolonged heavy drinking

---

[105] Ibid.

over longer periods of time can affect you in many different ways.[106]

Other Effects

Alcohol affects the parts of your brain that control judgment, concentration, coordination, behavior, and emotions. If you binge drink, you may be at greater risk of the following:

- becoming a victim of crime, for example, rape, domestic violence, mugging, or assault;
- being involved in antisocial or criminal behavior, for example, fights, domestic violence, vandalism, or theft;
- having an accident, for example, a road accident, fall, accident at work, or accidental fire;
- losing your job because of repeated absences or poor performance (think about the financial consequences);
- damaging relationships with family or friends.[107]

29. The following is adapted from the National Institute on Alcohol Abuse and Alcoholism and *Men's Health*:

---

[106] Ibid.
[107] Ibid.

Your Brain

Contrary to popular belief, alcohol doesn't actually kill your brain cells, says David Sack, MD, CEO of the addiction treatment company Elements Behavioral Health. But alcohol does alter levels of neurotransmitters, the chemical messengers that control your mood, perception, and behavior, he says.

Alcohol impairs brain areas such as the cerebellum—the control site for your balance and coordination—and your cerebral cortex, which is responsible for thinking, memory, and learning, says Kimberly S. Walitzer, PhD, deputy director of the University of Buffalo's Research Institute on Addictions.[108]

Plus, University of Michigan researchers found the amygdala—an area of the brain involved in fear and anger—showed less of a reaction to threatening faces after a single drink, potentially explaining why you're prone to risky behavior (such as fighting a bouncer) under the influence.[109]

---

[108] *Men's Health*, October 12, 2015.
[109] Ibid.

Your Skin

Sure, beer goggles may make other people appear hotter, but booze doesn't do your own mug many favors. Alcohol messes with your face, dilating blood vessels and making them more prone to breakage. This gives you bloodshot eyes and worsens a ruddy-skinned condition called rosacea, says dermatologist David E. Bank of Columbia Presbyterian Medical Center. Your heart pumps more fluid into surrounding tissues to balance out those alcohol-widened arteries and veins, leaving you with a bloated, puffy face.[110]

Your Muscles

Hit the gym as hard as you want, but if you hightail it to the bar afterward, you may never build bigger biceps. Alcohol tinkers with your hormonal and inflammatory responses to exercise, making it more difficult for your body to repair damaged proteins and build new ones (essential steps in getting ripped), according to a recent review in the journal *Sports Medicine*.

You'll compound this effect if you reach for a beer before a recovery snack or shake, says

---

[110] Ibid.

study author Matthew Barnes, PhD, of Massey University in New Zealand.

So, take the time to get some protein, carbohydrates, and nonboozy fluids into your system postworkout before cracking open your first cold one.[111]

Your Heart

Moderate drinking might protect your ticker because of the blood-vessel-relaxing polyphenols that alcohol contains or by raising your levels of HDL ("good" cholesterol), says researcher Kirsten Mehlig, PhD, of the University of Gothenburg in Sweden. But her recent study in the journal *Alcohol* suggests these effects may only benefit the 15 percent of the population with a certain genetic profile affecting HDL levels. It's too soon to recommend genetic testing to guide your alcohol consumption, she points out.

Meanwhile, those same two drinks per day can raise your risk of atrial fibrillation by 17 percent, according to a study in the *Journal of the American College of Cardiology*.[112]

---

[111] Ibid.

[112] Ibid.

This type of irregular heartbeat approximately quadruples your risk of having a stroke and triples your risk of heart failure.

Your Stomach

Just one night of bingeing—that's five drinks or more for guys in about two hours—increases what's called your gut permeability, according to University of Massachusetts Medical School researchers.

Harmful toxins and bacteria leak from your digestive system into your bloodstream, prompting a dangerous immune system response that can eventually lead to liver disease and other health problems.

At lower doses, alcohol irritates your stomach, increases acidity, and relaxes the muscle at the end of your esophagus, causing heartburn, Dr. Sacks says.[113]

Your Penis

Having as few as five drinks a week decreases your sperm count and percentage of healthy swimmers, perhaps by affecting levels of sex hormones such

---

[113]   Ibid.

as testosterone, Danish researchers recently reported in the journal *BMJ* (*British Medical Journal*) *Open*.

And while you may find a glass of vino sets the mood, anything more than that could wreck your performance in the bedroom, Dr. Sacks says.

Almost three-quarters of men with alcohol dependence have at least one sexual health issue, such as low desire, erectile dysfunction, or premature ejaculation, say Indian researchers.[114]

30. The following is from the *Telegraph*:

What Alcohol Does to Your Body after the Age of 40

Generally speaking, the older you get, the longer that alcohol stays in your system (i.e., metabolism).

If you're over 40 and live in Britain, the chances are you like a drink. A YouGov survey found "empty nester" mothers were at the forefront of the middle-aged drinking epidemic in Britain, with 28 per cent of women over 45 admitting they drank

---

[114] Ibid.

as much or more than their grown-up children. It's also the older generation—those 65 and over—[who] are most likely to drink on five consecutive nights each week. As the Chief Medical Officer Dame Sally Davies considers the current NHS drinking guidelines, experts are urging us to spare a thought not only to the short-term effects of alcohol on our brains, but also to the damage our drinking habits are doing to our bodies as we approach middle age.

A pioneering Danish study found that tee-totallers got pregnant much sooner than even very light "social" drinkers and they had a lower miscarriage rate.

"Alcohol affects just about every system because it's a small molecule that goes everywhere in the body," says Paul Wallace, emeritus professor of public health at University College London and medical director of the charity Drinkaware. "From the gut to the heart, the blood vessels to the skin, its effects are all pervasive." But why does it feel like the effects of drinking are so much worse post-40? "The organs that metabolize alcohol such as the liver and the stomach shrink as you get older, so alcohol stays in your system longer," says Dr Tony Rao, consultant old age psychiatrist at the South London and Maudsley NHS Foundation Trust. This could explain that wretched two-day hangover post-40. "Plus, the total fluid in the body is a lot less—we get more dehydrated as we get older—so because alcohol is distributed in blood which will be more concentrated, it won't be broken down as quickly as it would in the bloodstream of a 20 year old."

"Alcohol gets through the blood-brain barrier where it works as a depressant," says Professor Wallace. "We feel quite excited and stimulated when we drink because it's having a depressing effect on controlling behaviors such as judgement, self-monitoring, planning and reasoning," he says. It explains why what seemed like great idea the night before is not so much the morning after. "Over time this gives you a higher propensity to mood problems such as anxiety and depression." In his NHS clinic specializing in alcohol problems, Dr Rao sees people in their 60s with subtle alcohol related brain damage after a lifetime of casual drinking. "I always say to my patients[,] 'Your brain is affected a lot earlier than your liver,'" he says. "Before we see the cirrhosis[,] we see depression and problems with impulse control, moodiness, problems making complex decisions, say with finances and their children or spouses might say, 'Oh that's just so-and-so being a silly old bugger,' so the problems are missed. Good news is, the damage can be reversed after just six months of not drinking," he says.[115]

Fertility

A pioneering Danish study of thousands of couples who had discontinued contraception in order to conceive found that tee-totallers got pregnant much sooner than even very light "social" drinkers and they had a lower miscarriage rate. Even where couples resort to IVF, a US study found that moderate drinking (half a bottle of wine a week) was associated with an 18 per cent reduction in success rates for women. "For men, excessive alcohol

---

[115] *Telegraph*, November 8, 2019; Cheat Sheet, June 11, 2018; the *Sydney Morning Herald*, December 15, 2015.

consumption lowers testosterone levels and reduces sperm quality and quantity," says Dr. Gillian Lockwood, fertility specialist and medical director of Midland Fertility. "The 'sperm cycle' is 70 days, so the damaging effect of a serious binge may take a couple of months to improve, a more serious consideration for men over 40 whose sperm is already declining in quality."[116]

---

[116] Ibid.

Weight

Alcohol contains seven calories per gram, nearly the same as fat (9 calories per gram) and when you drink the body recognizes its by-products as toxins and chooses to break these down first over the nutrients in food, explains nutritionist Robert Hobson, co-author of *The Detox Kitchen Bible* (Bloomsbury). "When the body gets round to metabolizing the food, it may no longer require the calories, so they get stored as fat."

Studies also show that drinking can suppress the hormone leptin, which controls appetite which is why people can over eat when drinking. As a sugar source, alcohol raises insulin and turns on fat storage by increasing fatty deposits in the liver and, in middle age, excess can lead to fat storage around the stomach—a root cause of the classic "beer belly."[117]

31. *Plan ahead!*

---

[117] Ibid.

CHAPTER 8

Milk and Other Dairy Products

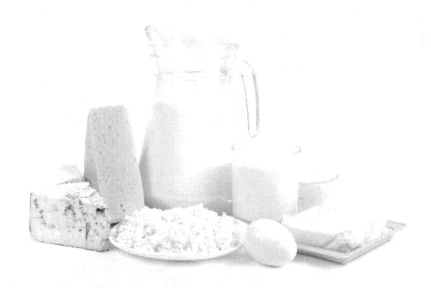

Milk, Cream, and Other Dairy Products

In many ways this is the hardest chapter to write because some people who like and use milk swear by it as one of the wonders of the world and a secret key to their health and wellness, both physically and mentally, whereas other profess the idea that milk is one of the worst things that you can put into your body. So, what do the experts and scientists say about milk?

In general, within *The Nutrient Diet*, I'm going to try to persuade you (with both data and my opinions and experiences) to try some practices and habits that you may not have tried before. Some of those practices will include actions and habits that I believe will be effective for you that you may not necessarily believe in or trust—which is why I provide data, research, studies, and information that I hope will help promote your beliefs in taking these actions, at least enough to give them a real try, even when it might go against some of your past experiences, instincts, and intuitions. Still, in some cases, I'm going to suggest that you go with your instincts based on your body's reactions to your actions. And, yes, this is based on my own experiences.

When looking back at my childhood, I recall that certain foods didn't necessarily sit well with me (with my skin, or my throat, or my stomach, or my head, and so forth). When I was as young as four to eight, both my mother and I got a sense about what those foods were. They included things such as milk and orange juice. As I went through several decades, and as my taste buds and allergies developed and matured, I noticed that while my allergies to certain things seemed to lessen, my allergies to some other things seemed to become greater. And then they would change again.

I'll also share with you that I was born over a month premature. I've always had bad allergies (i.e., allergic reactions to certain stimuli). When I was tested for allergies during college and during medical school, my reactions were so bad that they had to cease the tests. I was also sick all through anatomy during medical school and during many of my clinical clerkships (such as ER medicine and pediatrics—anything involving hospitals), which led me to take antihistamines and/or receive allergy shots.

Over the past four and a half decades, I've realized and accepted that I am allergic to some foods—and these, correspondingly, tend to mount an allergic, inflammatory response. These foods include the following: (1) milk, (2) some fruits such as melons, (3) white and red wine, and (4) certain vegetables, such as avocados. Regardless of what science, experts, studies, research, articles, dieticians, or physicians say about these foods, I avoid them because I trust myself, my body, and my body's responses and reactions to certain substances. For example, all the foods I just listed above make me produce phlegm, irritate my throat or other parts of my digestive tract, and overall just don't sit well with me (causing headaches or hot flashes, in the case of wines).

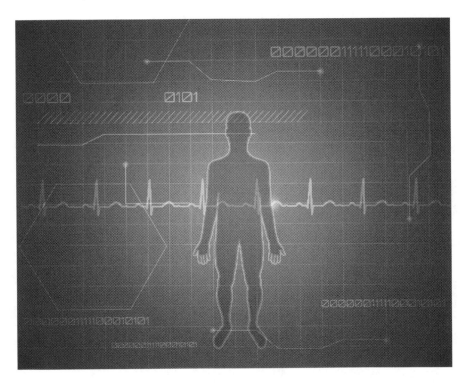

So, regardless of *anything* that I say, suggest, or promote in *The Nutrient Diet*, if a certain food makes you feel bad, if you have an inflammatory reaction to it, if it just doesn't sit right with you, or if it makes you sick, then don't consume it—regardless of anything anyone says. Now, I wouldn't use that advice for things like water. You need water. But when it comes to processed foods and other foods from which you can obtain the same or similar nutrients as other food to which you don't have negative reactions or responses, find an alternative that feels good to you, your body, and your overall feeling of wellness, health, and wholeness. If nothing else, learn to trust yourself, your body, your instincts, and your intuitions. After all, no one else on this planet has your combination of genes, gene expression, environmental experiences, reactions, and senses. Only you have that specific combination of locks and keys.

According to *Medical Daily*, the following are true regarding milk:

- It can help to lower blood glucose.
  According to a recent study, milk consumed with a high-carbohydrate breakfast could help lower blood glucose levels even after lunch. The effect was particularly strong with high-protein milk. Dairy milk naturally contains two high-quality proteins: whey (20 percent) and casein (80 percent). Their digestion leads to the release of gastric hormones that slow digestion and help increase feelings of fullness.[118]

- It provides calcium, vitamin D, and vitamin B$_{12}$. "Cow's milk on its own—without fortification—has 300 milligrams of calcium, which is 30 percent of the recommended daily allowance for most adults," said Dr. Amanda Powell of the Boston

---

[118] Sadhana Bharanidharan, "Is Drinking Milk Good for You? 3 Pros and Cons," Medical Daily, August 20, 2018, https://www.medicaldaily.com/drinking-milk-good-you-3-pros-and-cons-426975.

Medical Center. And when fortified, it can also provide a healthy dose of vitamin D, which is needed by the body for the absorption of calcium. "And, one cup of milk has half of the recommended daily allowance of B$_{12}$," Powell added.[119]

- It is recommended for growing children.
  The United States Department of Agriculture notes that the intake of dairy products is very important during the periods of childhood and adolescence. The often-cited reason is that calcium can benefit bone mass, which is still being built during this stage. Research has also suggested that children who drink cow's milk may grow up to be taller than their counterparts who drink nondairy substitutes.[120]

- It contains lactose, which can be harmful.
  The dairy sugar, known as lactose, cannot be digested and broken down by everyone's body. Those who are unable to digest milk properly suffer from what is known as lactose intolerance, which can cause symptoms such as gas, nausea, bloating, diarrhea, and cramps. If you are prone to these, experts recommend removing dairy from your diet to see whether the symptoms subside.

[119] Ibid.
[120] Ibid.

You can also see a doctor, who can confirm the diagnosis with the help of a lactose tolerance test, a hydrogen breath test, or a stool acidity test.[121]

- It can wreak havoc on your skin, causing acne. Acne is an inflammatory condition, says board-certified dermatologist Joshua Zeichner from Mount Sinai Hospital. And milk sourced from cows is capable of causing inflammation and triggering a breakout. Milk contains a hormone known as IGF-1, which is released by whey and casein. Not only is it similar to insulin in terms of structure, but also it can promote the formation of acne.[122]

- It has a lot more calories than you would expect. While high on nutrition, dairy milk is also high in calorie value—just one cup of 2 percent milk is said to contain about one hundred twenty calories. So even consuming one glass per meal would add up to three hundred sixty calories, which makes up 20 percent of the recommended caloric intake for the day. To cut down on consumption, consider drinking your coffee or tea every day without milk. Dr. Gail Cresci from the Cleveland Clinic recommends sticking to one glass of milk per day.

---

[121] Ibid.
[122] Ibid.

Here's my take based on this information: If you have a child who enjoys drinking milk and does not appear to have any aversions, reactions, or allergies to it, then, by all means, allow him or her to have it. It should be beneficial to his or her growth and development for about eighteen to twenty-four years. If your child doesn't like milk, or if he or she has an aversion, or reactions, or allergies to it, then seek other alternatives (almond milk, coconut milk, Silk, etc.). However, you as an adult should make the choice of whether or not to drink milk based on how well it sits with you and whether or not you enjoy it. If you choose whole milk, I wouldn't recommend more than one cup per day. In addition, keep in mind that the milk that you get from cows comes from what the cows have consumed. If those cows have been fed or exposed to pesticides or other chemicals, then those chemicals could be showing up in your milk.

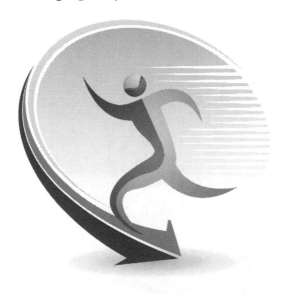

Also, recall that milk may contain insulin-like growth factor 1, which comes from whey and casein. IGF-1 is also called somatomedin C. According to UpToDate, insulin-like growth factor-1 is a hormone that functions as the major mediator of growth hormone–stimulated somatic growth, as well as a mediator of growth hormone–independent anabolic responses in many cells and tissues.[123] Here's the reason why milk is good for children in general and good for adults in certain circumstances: IGF-1 exerts its effects via activation of the IGF-1 receptor. This receptor is widely distributed, which enables blood-transported IGF-1 to coordinate balanced growth among multiple tissues and organs. In contrast, autocrine/paracrine IGF-1 can stimulate local, unbalanced growth independently of systemic growth hormone. Examples of this type of growth regulation are wound healing and growth of the contralateral kidney after unilateral nephrectomy.[124]

According to Healthline, here's what you need to know about milk:

---

[123] David R. Clemmons, Peter J. Snyder, and Kathryn A. Martin, "Physiology of Insulin-Like Growth Factor 1," UpToDate, https://www.uptodate.com/contents/physiology-of-insulin-like-growth-factor-1.
[124] Ibid.

Milk is considered a whole food. It provides eighteen of the twenty-two essential nutrients.[125]

Nutrient	Amount per 1 cup (244 grams) of whole milk	Percentage of recommended daily amount (RDA)
Calcium	276 mg	28 percent
Folate	12 mcg	3 percent
Magnesium	24 mg	7 percent
Phosphorus	205 mg	24 percent
Potassium	322 mg	10 percent
Vitamin A	112 mcg	12.5 percent
Vitamin B_{12}	1.10 mcg	18 percent
Zinc	0.90 mg	11 percent
Protein	7–8 grams (casein and whey)	16 percent

Milk also provides iron, selenium, vitamin B_6, vitamin E, vitamin K, niacin, thiamin, and riboflavin.

Fat content varies. Whole milk contains more fat than other types of milk, as follows:

- saturated fats, 4.5 grams
- unsaturated fats, 1.9 grams
- cholesterol, 24 milligrams (mg)[126]

[125] Noreen Iftikhar, "Pros and Cons of Drinking Cow's Milk," Healthline, May 11, 2020.
[126] Ibid.

Appetite Control

Drinking milk hasn't been linked to weight gain or obesity, and it may help curb appetite. A 2013 study of forty-nine people showed that dairy helped people feel fuller and reduced how much fat they ate overall. Some studies have shown that full-fat dairy intake is associated with lower body weight. And some have shown that dairy intake, in general, may prevent weight gain.

Diabetes Prevention and Heart Health

Several studies have found that drinking milk may help prevent type 2 diabetes in adults. This may be because milk proteins improve your blood sugar balance. Milk fat may help raise levels of HDL (good) cholesterol. Having healthy HDL cholesterol levels may prevent heart disease and stroke. Additionally, milk is a good source of potassium. This mineral helps regulate blood pressure. Pastured or grass-fed cows make milk with more omega-3 fatty acids and conjugated linoleic acid. These fats help protect heart and blood vessel health.[127]

Problems caused by milk, according to Dr. Noreen Iftikhar, are as follows:

---

[127]   Ibid.

Acne

A 2016 study found that teenagers with acne drank higher amounts of low-fat or skim milk than those without acne. Dairy may also trigger adult acne. Other studies have linked acne to skim and low-fat milk. This may be due to milk's influence on certain hormones, including insulin and insulin-like growth factor-1. More research is needed to explore the connection between diet and acne.[128]

Other Skin Conditions

Eczema

Some foods may worsen eczema, including milk and dairy, according to a clinical review. However, a 2018 study found that pregnant and breastfeeding women who added a probiotic to their diet reduced their child's risk for eczema and other food-related allergic reactions.[129]

Rosacea

Dairy may also be a trigger food for some adults with rosacea. On the other hand, a recent study suggests that dairy may actually have a positive effect on rosacea.[130]

---

[128] Ibid.

[129] Ibid.

[130] Ibid.

Allergies

Up to 5 percent of children have a milk allergy, some experts estimate. Milk can cause skin reactions, such as eczema, and gut symptoms, such as colic, constipation, and diarrhea.[131]

Other serious reactions include anaphylaxis (shock), wheezing, difficulty breathing, and bloody stool.

Children may grow out of a milk allergy. Adults may also develop a milk allergy.

Bone Fractures

Drinking three or more glasses of milk per day may increase the risk of bone fractures in women. Research found that this may be due to a sugar called D-galactose in milk. However, the study did explain that further research is needed before dietary recommendations are made. Another study showed that bone fractures in older adults, the result of osteoporosis, are highest in areas that consume more dairy, animal protein, and calcium.[132]

---

[131] Ibid.
[132] Ibid.

Cancer

Excess calcium from milk and other foods may increase the risk of prostate cancer. Milk sugars may be linked to a slightly higher risk of ovarian cancer.[133]

Lactose Intolerance

Cow's milk has a higher amount of lactose than milk from other animals. A 2015 review estimates 65 percent to 70 percent of the world's population has some form of lactose intolerance. Most people with this condition can safely add small amounts of dairy to their diet.[134]

The good news is that if you decide to keep milk in your diet despite all these reported possible reactions, responses, and outcomes, you can choose an alternative to cow's milk.

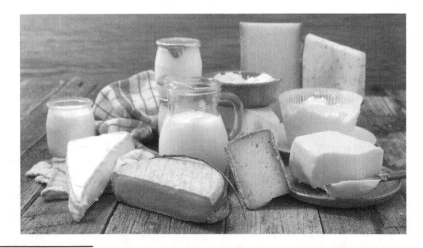

---

[133] Ibid.
[134] Ibid.

Alternatives to Milk

Cow's milk alternatives for infants and toddlers with milk protein allergies include the following:

Type	Pros	Cons
Breastfeeding	Best source of nutrition	Not all women can breastfeed
Amino acid formulas	Least likely to cause an allergic reaction	hypoallergenic formulas; produced with enzymes to break down milk proteins; processing may damage other nutrients
Soy-based formulas	Fortified to be nutritionally complete	Processing may damage other nutrients
		Some may develop an allergy to soy

Plant- and nut-based milks that are suitable for individuals who are lactose intolerant or vegan include the following:

Type	Pros	Cons
Soy milk	Contains similar amount of proteins	Contains plant estrogens and half the carbs and fats of whole milk hormones
Almond milk	Low fat; high calcium (if enriched); high vitamin E	Low protein; contains phytic acid (which hinders mineral absorption)
Coconut milk	Low calories and carbs; half the fat	No protein; high saturated fats
Oat milk	Lower in fat; high fiber	High carbs; low protein
Cashew milk	Low calories and fat	Low protein; fewer nutrients
Hemp milk	Low calories and carbs; high essential fatty acids	Low protein (though more than other plant-based milks)
Rice milk	Low fat	Low protein and nutrients; high carbs
Quinoa milk	Low fat, calories, and carbs	Low protein

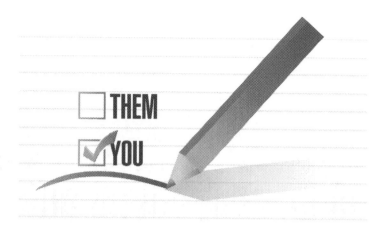

Dr. Iftikhar's Takeaways

✓ Milk is naturally packed with essential nutrients in a convenient and accessible form. Drinking milk is particularly important for children. It may help you and your child maintain good health.

✓ Milk nutrition varies. Milk from grass-fed or pastured cows provides more beneficial fats and higher amounts of some vitamins.

✓ More research is needed on the amount of milk that is most beneficial and on the effects of antibiotics and artificial hormones given to dairy cows.

✓ It's best to choose organic milk from cows that are free of growth hormones.

✓ Milk alternatives can also be part of a healthy, balanced diet.[135]

Here's my take on this information: Again, when it comes to processed foods and other foods from which you can obtain the same or similar nutrients as other food to which you don't have negative reactions or responses, find an alternative that feels good to you and your body and that enhances your overall feelings of wellness, health, and wholeness. If nothing else, learn to trust yourself, your body, your instincts, and your intuitions. After all, no one else on this planet has your combination of genes, gene expression, environmental experiences, reactions, or senses. Only you have that specific combination of locks and keys. And remember, when you are consuming products from animals, you are also consuming much of what they have consumed, pesticides, hormones, chemicals, and all. If a certain type of milk or other dairy product agrees with you, then indulge in it. But keep it down to small portions; don't overindulge. If you are dieting, it may help you to choose an alternative to cow's milk until your weight is where you want it to be.

---

[135] Noreen Iftikhar, "Pros and Cons of Drinking Cow's Milk," Healthline, May 11, 2020.

CHAPTER 9

The Basics of Vitamins and Minerals

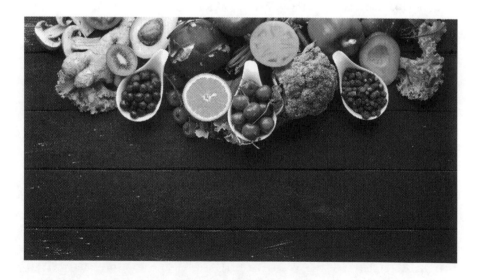

It's so *simple*, yet it's so *complex*! You *are* what you eat! But soon the question becomes "What are you eating?" That question is a bit more difficult to answer since very few of us *really, truly* know what's in the food that we buy and consume. That is, unless you plant and grow your own food or you know exactly where your food comes from (and, hence, how it was planted and grown).

So many of us have such busy, on-the-go lives that we don't take the time (or assume the responsibility) to know exactly what we're eating *and* ensure that we're getting the right allocation of nutrients daily. It's *not* easy. However, it is doable!

A few of the dietary deficiencies that may be associated with conditions that can have an effect on your daily mental health, well-being, and emotionality are as follows: (1) low vitamin C (ascorbate/ascorbic acid); (2) low magnesium (Mg+); (3) low vitamin D_2, D_3, or D_4 (cholecalciferol); (4) low iron (Fe+); (5) low iodine (I–); (6) low calcium (Ca+); (7) low vitamin A (retinol/beta carotene); (8) low vitamin B_1 (thiamine) or B_2 (riboflavin); (9) low vitamin B_3 (niacin); (10) low vitamin B_4 (biotin) (a.k.a. vitamin H); (11) low vitamin B_5 (pantothenic acid); (12) low vitamin B_6 (pyridoxine) (a.k.a. vitamin M) or vitamin B_9 (folate/folic acid); (13) low vitamin B_{12} (cobalamin); (14) low potassium (K+); (15) low vitamin E (tocopherol); (16) low vitamin K_1 or K_2; (17) low omega-3 fatty acids; (18) low choline; (19) low ferritin; (20) low copper (Cu+); (21) low chromium; (22) low serotonin; (23) low dopamine; (24) low GABA; (25) low melatonin; (26) low glutamate; (27) low tryptophan;

(28) low manganese (Mn); (29) low selenium (Se); (30) low sodium (Na+); and (31) low zinc (Zn+).

In general, vitamins are broken into two general categories:

- those that are fat soluble and are therefore stored in the body (vitamins A, D, E, and K [ADEK]) and
- those that are water soluble and are therefore *not* stored in the body and must be consumed *daily* (the vast majority of the B vitamins, and vitamin C).

If a vitamin is fat-soluble, it simply means that it's a vitamin your body can store in an organ and/or tissue (such as your liver).

Then there are the major minerals: iron, copper, calcium, manganese, selenium, and sodium. Since the vitamins and minerals in your body (in general) work together, a shortage of one can lead to dysfunction associated with another. Generally speaking, you can develop symptoms for either a deficiency or a surplus of fat-soluble vitamins. However, as long as you're hydrated, you will only develop symptoms from a water-soluble vitamin if you have a deficiency.

If you don't ensure that you're getting each and every one of these on a weekly (fat-soluble vitamins) or daily basis (water-soluble vitamins) (depending on the type of vitamin or mineral), then you should be supplementing your diet on a *consistent* basis. Not doing so can lead to a number of mental health, emotional, mood-associated, and psychiatric problems.

In fact, many individuals who have been diagnosed with a psychiatric disorder may, indeed, simply suffer from a nutrient deficiency!

Then the psychotropic agent (i.e., medication) that has been prescribed ostensibly to treat the problem may cause additional deficiencies and side effects—leading to a downhill avalanche of cascading symptoms and dilemmas.

However, don't take my word for it. Researchers have been suggesting for decades that diet is *essential* to optimum mental health. However, in the past, there were few clinical trials available to agree with them. But such is not the case now.

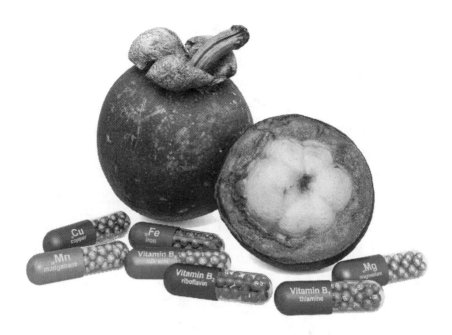

I could provide you with a great deal of sound data regarding the human body's need for the basic nutrients and their building blocks (neurotransmitters, carrier molecules, amino acids, transport proteins, fats, vitamins, minerals, etc.), including a recent study that illustrated the power of nutrition to lift depressive symptoms. However, there are many resources available on the internet (including clinical trial data and other studies) to illustrate this. These resources are readily available to everyone these days. All you have to do is type in the name of the amino acid, the protein, the type of fat, the vitamin, the mineral, or other type of substance, and more information than you ever wanted to know will present itself.

Instead of rehashing that information, I'd like to present you with some time-tested general principles regarding vitamins, minerals, and other essential nutrients in order to help you make better selection, buying, and consumption decisions:

- As a general rule, if it's cheap, then it's probably not very good (given the lack of quality controls, the potency, the sourcing, the testing, etc.).
- Go to a trusted, informed, up-to-date, root-cause-oriented, physiology-based healthcare provider who knows what he or she is talking about when it comes to vitamins, minerals, and other essential nutrients.
- Don't trust just anybody's advice or guidance.
- Get a good trustworthy book on nutrition from a highly qualified author.
- Get a good trustworthy book on herbs and alternative medicine / alternative healthcare from a highly qualified author (such as C. Normal Shealy's *Illustrated Encyclopedia of Healing Remedies and Alternative Healthcare: A Comprehensive Guide to Therapies and Remedies*).
- Take vitamins and minerals early in the morning with breakfast.
- When trying herbal products, institute one thing at a time (i.e., for mental sharpness, first try gingko biloba for four weeks and *then* try gotu

kola for four weeks—don't initiate both at the same time).

- Look at all the ingredients and percentages of each ingredient on the back of the label.
- Avoid formulations that lack an ingredients label.
- Look out for added caffeine sources in designer multivitamin formulations, as you may already be receiving plenty of caffeine from another source.
- Drink lots of water with your vitamins and nutrients.
- Take vitamins and minerals with your breakfast, not by themselves.
- Be careful about taking over 100 percent of the US RDA (recommended daily allowance) when it comes to fat-soluble vitamins (i.e., vitamins A, D, E, and K). That could lead to psychiatric symptoms, among other things.
- Understand that while fat-soluble vitamins and some B vitamins make stay in your system for days, weeks, or months, other vitamins (primarily the water-soluble vitamins) need to be taken daily.
- Do *not* substitute vitamins, minerals, supplements, shakes, or formulations for meals. These should augment your regular dietary intake, not replace it.
- Do *not* take vitamins on an empty stomach.
- Check with your trusted, informed, up-to-date, root-cause-oriented, physiology-based healthcare

provider before starting a new formulation or supplement.

- Check with your trusted, informed, up-to-date, root-cause-oriented, physiology-based healthcare provider prior to trying new diets.
- Avoid a fat-free diet. Your brain is made up of fats, and your body requires fats to create hormones. In fact, cholesterol is the molecular *backbone* of all your body's hormones. The key is to get the healthier, more-high-density fats from natural sources (e.g., avocados, fresh fish, nuts).
- Remember that adequate, consistent nutrition is the *basis of health*. There are no permanent substitutes for it if you desire to live a full, balanced, healthy, and purposeful life.
- Invest in educating yourself about nutrition, health, and lifestyle choices. You may find that what you discover is different from what uninformed, well-meaning friends, relatives, and coworkers might tell you.
- Trust how you feel, trust your body, and develop strong instincts regarding what works for you and what doesn't—in concert with advice and wisdom from a trusted, informed, up-to-date, root-cause-oriented, physiology-based healthcare provider.

Consistency is key!

CHAPTER 10

Snacks

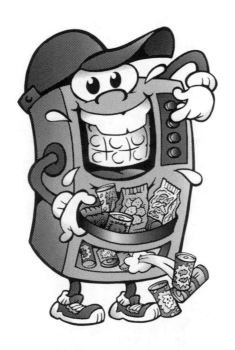

Snacks and Snacking

It should come as absolutely no surprise to you that snacking can completely undermine a diet, a weight loss plan, a weight-management effort, or a health-driven lifestyle. However, it may surprise you that there are dozens of strategies that people use to control and monitor their snacking habits that are simple, easy, doable, and nondrastic.

Thankfully, when it comes to snacking, strategy is key!

So, let's get started with snacking.

I'm going to present my top-ten list for snaking. I'll also be sharing with you how to snack successfully and what to do if following my advice doesn't work for you the first time around.

1. You must have a vision, a goal, a plan, and a strategy.

    In general, this is dieting, weight loss, weight management, and healthy lifestyle 101. If you want to be successful in anything, then you have to have a goal, a plan, and a strategy. Again, for anything that you want to be successful at, even if you're already good at it (innately or after a great deal of practice and repetition), you need a goal, a plan, and a strategy.

    ▪ Your vision should be an ideal but realistic version of yourself and your weight. It should be encompassing of the lifestyle you wish to lead and should reflect a lifestyle that you have the ability to maintain on a long-term basis.

- Your goals should be incremental in nature. For instance, if you've gained fifty pounds during the past twelve to twenty-four months (i.e., you went from weighing 185 pounds to weighing 235 pounds), then while your final weight loss goal might be one hundred eighty-five pounds, your immediate weight goal should be to lose five pounds during the next two weeks. Your focus should be primarily on the incremental goal, not the long-term goal, because incremental goals are more realistic. But you should be visualizing the long-term goal. You need to do both simultaneously.

- Your daily, weekly, and monthly plans should be based on three to five small meals per day. Your plans should include snacks and meals and should indicate how much of each you are permitted to consume to stay within range. Your plans for snacks should be as specific as your plans for meals.

- Your strategy should be specific, goal-driven, and reward-based. When you reach your goals, you should reward yourself at the end of the day, or with tiny rewards at intervals throughout the day (e.g., every three hours or every four hours). Your strategy should be specific yet flexible in nature. And it should be in real time. For instance, if it's Thursday and you know that you have plans for a calorie-rich dinner on Friday night, then use that fact to help motivate you to eat and snack wisely up until that Friday night meal. Then, portion out that Friday meal so you have two small meals or snacks for the next day (or one for Saturday and one for Sunday). When I go out for surf and turf on Friday night, I eat about one-third of my meal, and then I eat the other two-thirds on two separate occasions over the next two days. That way, I'm rewarding myself for the entire weekend for my strategic behaviors on Thursday and Friday!

2. Plan your snacks ahead of time.

Know the approximately calorie count of your snacks.

Control the portion size of your snacks using ziplock bags.

If you desire snacks that aren't so healthy, either pair them with healthier snacks (which is the principle of bargaining and compromising) or have healthier snacks in between.

Have at least one cup of water with your snacks.

- Gradually increase the amount of water and decrease the amount of the snack during snack times.
- Use your snacks to decrease the sizes of your breakfast, lunch, and dinner meals.

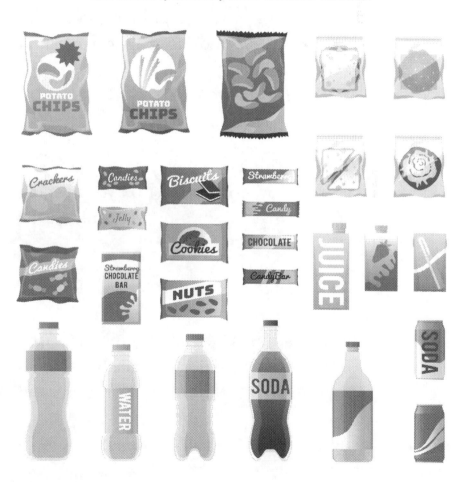

3. Always have multiple choices ahead of time.

   - Prepack your snacks.
   - Use small portions of your favorite foods as snacks (e.g., one-sixth of a Reuben sandwich, two hundred calories of lasagna (two bites or two spoonsful, etc.).
   - Consider things such as granola bars, trail mix, almonds, jerky, dried fruit, carrots, and celery sticks.
   - Gradually migrate from less-healthy snacks to more-healthy snacks.

4. Don't snack on things that you already know you don't like or enjoy, because later on you're going to go back to what you originally desired in the first place.

   - Instead, create tiny portions of foods that you like and/or enjoy.
   - Also use online snacking groups for snack ideas (for instance, the bars made by 2 Moms [Google Search "2 Moms"] are delicious and healthy).
   - Post your snack ideas online to help reinforce you snacking behaviors.

5. Determine what type of snacker you are.

   - Are you a stress/nervousness/anxiety snacker?
   - Are you a muncher?
   - Are you a social snacker, that is, someone who snacks when there is company around? Is such snacking a part of your cultural identity and/or practices?

6. Enlist resources and other people to help hold you accountable.

   - Let others around you know what you are doing so they can assist in keeping you accountable.
   - Get a snacking app on your phone so you can keep track of the calories you consume.
   - Get a snacking partner through an online community or a mobile application.
   - Create homemade snack recipes that you can share online.

7. Make a list of what snacks you like. Have a variety of snack choices available. Availability, choices, and options are everything.

   Avoid snacks that you don't like. Eating undesirable snacks at the beginning of your weight loss program won't help promote a new behavior pattern.

8. Use your snack list to find alternatives and similar snacks that are equally good and satisfying for you but won't cause you to gain weight or break your diet plan.

- Compromise and balance to make snacking work for you (e.g., pair a lemon pepper chicken wing with a celery stick).
- Look for snacks that have anti-inflammatory properties.
- Look for snacks with fiber.
- Consider smoothies.

9. Join a healthy lifestyle group that will help you to find the best snacks for you. There are so many of these. Here are just a few:

- SnackNation.com
- WorkWeekLunch.com
- RealSimple.com
- SammiBrondo.com
- SnackSafely.com
- SparkPeople.com

10. Exercise and perform energy-requiring activities *around* your meals and snack times.

CHAPTER 11

Meal Planning and Meal Spacing

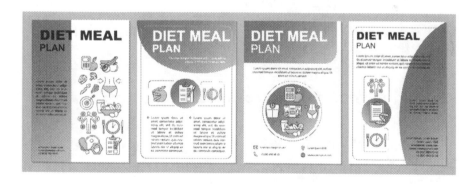

Meal planning, meal strategies, and meal spacing are keys to a healthy, balanced, and sustainable lifestyle because they are building blocks to behavior and are important to behavioral triggers and how your DNA expresses itself. Your hypothalamus, pituitary gland, gut hormones, neurotransmitters, and enzymes control your body's responses to food. They help to determine your triggers for hunger and for eating. So, if you can help to train them to be active in a way that is consistent with the body and lifestyle that you desire, instead of the body and lifestyle that you've had and currently have, then you will be successful with regard to your nutritional goals.

If you want to create a new set of behaviors that are *sustainable*, then you have to recruit your body to work with you to create them. Meal planning, meal strategies, and meal spacing are the keys to doing that.

So, what guidelines for meal planning, meal strategies, and meal spacing should you use to manage and/or control your weight and create the lifestyle you desire? Well, here's the list:

1. Plan your meals weeks to months ahead of time.

   - The key to what you will do at the present moment is what you did or didn't plan earlier, and the key to what you will do tomorrow is to plan today (or earlier).
   - If you fail to plan your meals ahead of time, then you're going to default to your existing and previous behaviors. These are called automatic responses and learned reactions. In order to prevent things from happening automatically, you have to plan and execute a new behavior *before* the old behavior even

has an opportunity to express itself. That's called being preemptive and proactive. Being *preemptive* and *proactive* prevents your cells, neurotransmitters, and hormones, and other expressions of your DNA, from doing what they've been taught to do by you automatically.

- Plan your meals for the week on the weekend (at least by the weekend prior to the week), and prepare and package your meals during the weekend so that you won't have to worry about it when mealtime arrives during the week.

- Try to plan meals that are relatively easy to heat up and eat so it's not a pain to get them ready when it's time to eat.

- Ziploc® gallon, quart and sandwich bags and multiple sizes of containers so that you can store your meals in the refrigerator and the freezer.

2. Plan your meals with your personality in mind.

- Make your meal plans realistic but optimistic.
- Don't prepare meals that you know ahead of time you won't like or eat.
- Plan your meals creatively and with variety in mind. Unless you're a person who truly enjoys having the same thing over and over,

every day of the week, please plan a variety of offerings.

- Have a variety of proteins in your meal plans if you enjoy them. If you're open to fish, then include a variety of fishes (salmon, cod, trout, tuna).
- Have a variety of vegetables available as well. Cut them up and store them in containers and bags just as you do with your fish, chicken breasts, etc.
- Get a set of easy recipe cards to help guide your meals.
- Have the spices you use (Italian, Asian, Creole, etc.) and enjoy in your foods.
- Get the right oils for cooking your foods (coconut oil, grape-seed oil, etc.).
- At least in the beginning, plan out meals that are easy and quick. I use the fifteen-minute rule: If it can't be removed from the freezer or refrigerator, seasoned, and cooked within fifteen minutes, then it doesn't make the list for a weekday meal.
- When in doubt, *simplicity* should be your highest goal.
- Plan your beverages just as you plan the rest of your meal.

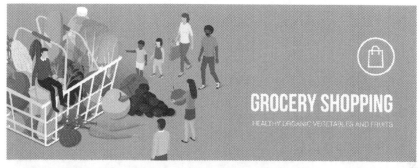

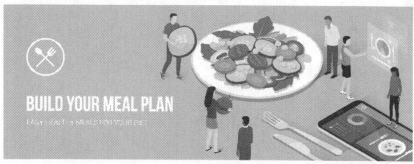

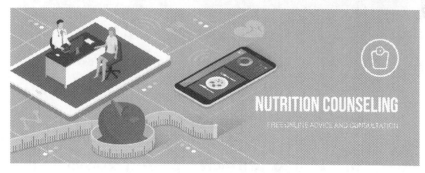

3. Implement good meal and eating strategies.

- *Always* have the ingredients to make a salad in your refrigerator—even if you don't use them. At this point, it's more important to establish new eating behaviors than it is for you to save money or conserve food.

- It should never be a choice between your meal planning and saving money. After all of this [considering the costs of chronic health conditions, medical office visits, tests, etc.] is said and done, you're going to save the money in the end anyway—while lowering your health risks for a host of medical conditions, including diabetes, hypertension, obesity, and metabolic syndrome.
- *Always* have fruits and nuts that you enjoy on standby.
- Until you have significantly reduced your portion sizes (which may take weeks to months), do *not* try to eat everything on your plate. It's a very bad idea, and it will thwart your weight loss efforts every single time because *sight* is the biggest trigger for eating. In fact, it's much easier to cook a meal that will last for two meal sessions and then eat only half of it for dinner, having the other half for lunch or dinner the next day or the day after that.
- Prepare your meals with creativity and variety, and seek outside sources for recipes. There are no shortages of smartphone apps, websites, or television shows showing how to cook healthy, delicious, simple, quick, and easy meals on a daily basis.

- Change your cooking and eating habits by interacting with others. Join meal, diet, lifestyle, and nutrition groups to help keep yourself excited and motivated about establishing and *maintaining* the lifestyle behaviors that you are creating. Also consider creating accountability partners who will help influence you during your troughs.

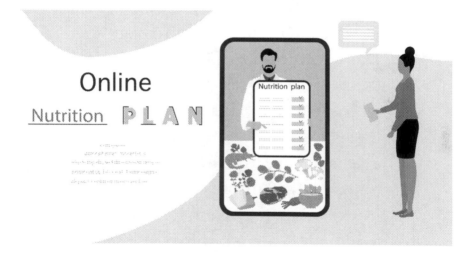

- Allow yourself to cheat occasionally. By occasionally, I mean no more than three times per week. You can help stick to this limit by creating cheat cards. Life and lifestyles should entail a degree of flexibility, compromise, and *fun*. After all, if you're being consistent, then the cheat sessions (as long as they are not over-the-top or extravagant) won't make that much of a difference.

- Have a calorie count in mind for your meals each day and a daily total. I shoot for between one thousand and fifteen hundred calories. Discover what works for you. Most diet and nutrition apps have calculators that will help you with your calorie goals and objectives.
- Use technology to help you meet your goals, objectives, and ambitions, but don't let these things control you. Just like with your phone, use it to help you, not control you.
- Don't be afraid to fail sometimes. Fear of failure is the *biggest* reason most people fail with their diet plans or fail to begin in the first place.
- You don't have to reinvent the wheel. Use the resources that are at your disposal.
- Don't boil foods, except for chicken. Boiling foods, in general, removes many of the elements that your body needs. Instead, learn from the Asian culture and other cultures that tend to stir-fry and/or sauté their foods.
- Use this as an opportunity to find a *balance* between eating for nutrition and eating for enjoyment. In general, you need to enjoy what you're eating. However, at the same time, every meal can't be like a birthday celebration. Celebratory meals are special because they are rare. If every meal became celebratory in

terms of the calorie count and composition, then you would spoil your mind, body, and spirit. That's not a healthy lifestyle.

- Use seasonings instead of salt to make your meals tastier. And note that, historically, salt has been used as a substitute for seasonings because the seasonings either weren't available or were too expensive to use on a daily basis. That isn't the case anymore. So, stop eating like it is the case. The same is true for fat.

- Teach yourself how to bake, stir-fry, and sauté foods instead of frying or boiling them. If you fry your foods in lots of grease/oil, then you're infusing them with a great many calories. If you boil them (such as boiling vegetables), then you're removing many of the important nutrients. As a general rule, if you boil something, if the water starts to take on the pigments from the foods, then you've overboiled it—because many of those nutrients are stored within those pigments.

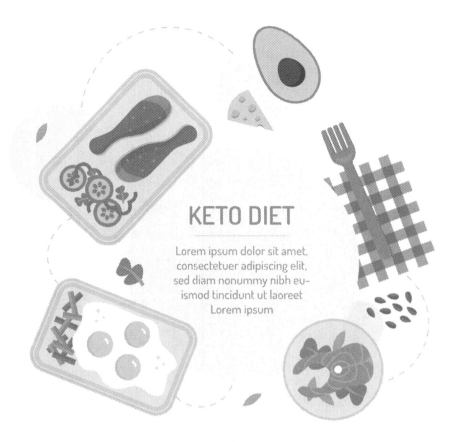

KETO DIET

Lorem ipsum dolor sit amet,
consectetuer adipiscing elit,
sed diam nonummy nibh eu-
ismod tincidunt ut laoreet
Lorem ipsum

4. As noted above, find a *balance* between eating for nutrition and eating for enjoyment. Balance is the key to lifestyle choices and behaviors. And balance is discovered, created, and negotiated.

5. If you get stuck, go to your resources. That's why they are there. Proactivity prevents reactivity!

6. Consider hiring a coach (even if only for a few weeks) to help you create, establish, and instill new eating behaviors.

7. Share your eating goals with coworkers, friends, and relatives so that you're actually recruiting them to hold you accountable, as well as influencing them to change their own behaviors.

8. If something isn't working, don't give up. Instead, be creative and come up with a different strategy for achieving the same goal.

9. Say positive affirmations before and after your meals, and plan to eat healthier desserts (such as half a cup of low-fat, low-sugar ice cream or sherbet) to reward yourself.

10. Do allow reasonable cheats and more of your favorite meals on weekends.

CHAPTER 12

Physical Activity and Exercise

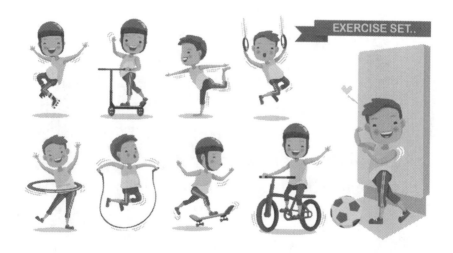

I'm not going to go into a great depth in this chapter, but I would like to provide some general advice, recommendations, and concepts regarding physical activity, as follows:

1. Exercise, physical activity, and sports are half the key to activating the genes that you need to create a healthy weight, maintain a healthy weight, and

establish a lifestyle that is a calculated but flexible, creating a compromise between your genes (i.e., your DNA) and your desires.

2. While your diet and nutrition practices and habits are key activators of gene expression and activity, exercise and muscular activity are just as important because they have a huge influence on the neurotransmitters that help influence how you feel, think, and behave.

3. Don't try to engage in exercises and activities that you genuinely don't like, unless someone else is willing to be your partner in learning to enjoy that activity. It's much easier and more sustainable to maximize the activities that you genuinely embrace and enjoy. For instance, if you enjoy bowling, then make that a part of your lifestyle.

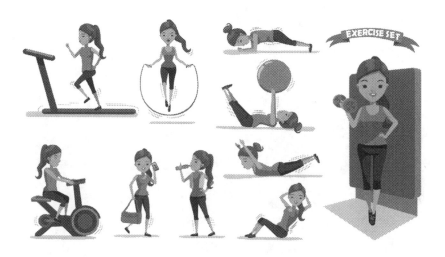

4. Use exercise and physical activity to help flush your system by drinking water during and following your workouts.

5. Plan and organize your physical activities just as you do your meals and snacks.

6. If you're new to or are reestablishing a physical activity habit, then use rewards to keep yourself motivated.

7. As with other habits and rituals, find and maintain accountability partners.

8. Say positive affirmations and mantras before and during your workouts.

9. Keep it simple. Please don't start out by trying to jog ten miles a day if it's been three years since

you last worked out, went to a gym, or jogged. Start small, and build from there. If you don't, then you're going to either overwhelm yourself or fail to live up to the unrealistic expectations that you've set.

10. Be creative, and use technology to help you. Also consider group activities such as yoga, cycling, aerobics, and team sports. Use music to make the time go by while you burn calories and create behaviors.

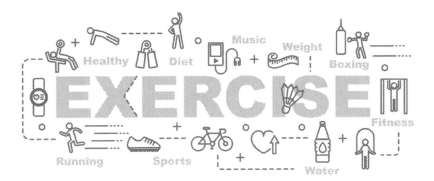

CHAPTER 13

Meditation and Hypnosis

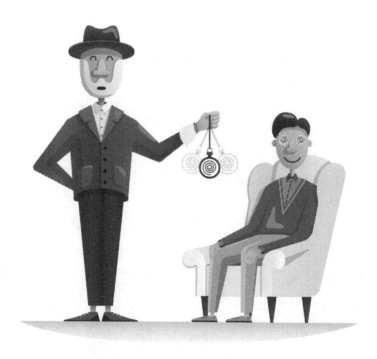

What is the *purpose* of hypnosis, and what can it be used for? Before we get to that, we should answer the question "What is hypnosis?"

I'm often asked what hypnosis is and how is it helpful. Hypnosis is a tool that helps people to achieve a state of consciousness that allows them to receive more information and to give out more information. It is a deeper, more relaxed state of consciousness where more barriers are broken and a person's conscious defenses are lowered. Once a hypnotic state has been induced, positive suggestions, messages, affirmations, thoughts, and ideas can be inserted to which the person will be much more receptive when not in the hypnotic state. This allows the person's subconscious mind to accept and absorb words, thoughts, ideas, and affirmations that he or she might normally reject if he or she were in a conscious state of mind (because so many defenses would be up).

What Does Hypnosis Allow?

The hypnotic state allows access to thoughts and feelings that have been buried because they may be too painful to deal with on a conscious level. These thoughts and feelings might include past hurts, rejections, painful experiences, traumatic experiences, and other repressed feelings and thoughts.

Hypnosis can be used to uncover thoughts and feelings that may have been forgotten or that have never been allowed to travel into consciousness because they may be too painful to take, experience, or relive.

What Is the Purpose of Hypnosis, and What Are Defense Mechanisms?

Much of the purpose of using hypnosis is to move past the defense mechanisms we have set up unconsciously to protect our views of ourselves, our loved ones, our beliefs, our belief systems, our desires, other people and of the world.

Our minds are very proactive and reactive when it comes to protecting us from things that might damage our well-being or else challenge the security we feel about the world around us. Because of this, defense mechanisms may become very complex and intricate. And they often elude us. One of the most common defense mechanisms is denial. It's common because it's *simple* and *easy*. Just deny what will challenge, damage, or interfere with your current views of society, people, and the world—which is thought to protect your present view of the world. It's actually a logical defense mechanism. The problem is that it fails to deal with reality and prevents you from growing, maturing, and evolving as a person. Another reason it's a very common defense mechanism is that it requires very little energy or thought. Other common defense mechanisms that you may have heard of include repression, reaction formation, sublimation, and rationalization. You tend to see repression and sublimation with people who have had to deal with repeated physical or psychological trauma. And you tend to see rationalization a lot in politics.

What Is the Relationship between Hypnosis and Fears and Anxieties?

Regardless of the defense mechanism or the reasons for its existence, hypnosis is a good tool for getting past any defense mechanism. It can also help calm fears and anxieties. For instance, many people have said that some people actually fear being successful. However, that's not the full story. People who are said to fear success don't usually fear success; what they usually fear is failure.

Hypnosis can be used to help eliminate fears and belief systems that prevent us from growing and maturing in ways that allow us to reach our goals and achieve success.

Hypnosis can all be used to delete limiting beliefs and adjust constraining belief systems.

What Hypnosis Is Not

Hypnosis does not involve mesmerizing people into doing things that they otherwise would object to doing. The words and phrases uttered during a hypnosis session should be well thought out, highly specific, and carefully configured and constructed so they do no harm. If they are not well thought out, then they can actually do more harm than good. That's why you should not trust just anyone to perform hypnosis on you or provide you with hypnotherapy.

The Role of Hypnosis in Weight Loss and Weight-Management Activities

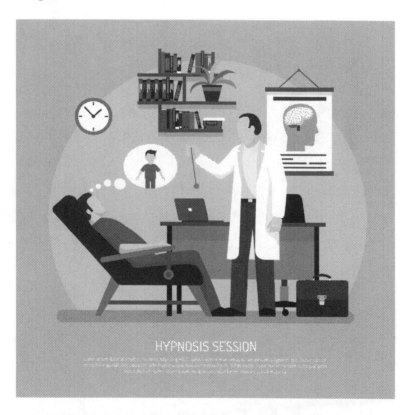

HYPNOSIS SESSION

Hypnosis is a great tool for dieting, weight loss, weight management, motivation, and lifestyle management because it can be used to change some of the limiting beliefs that may be subconsciously keeping you from being your best you. Hypnosis can also be used to get at some of the underlying causes of overeating, obesity, and poor lifestyle choices, such as stress, anxiety, worry, perfectionism, exhaustion, confidence, self-esteem, and trauma. Remember, overweightness and obesity are just symptoms of a larger issue. If you fail to chip away or eliminate the root cause(s), then the poor habits, the disadvantageous choices, and the weight will return.

How to Choose a Competent and Highly Qualified Hypnotherapist

If you are interested in trying hypnosis out of general curiosity, or if you're seeking hypnosis to help deal with a specific problem (such as depression, anxiety, poor self-confidence, insecurity, lack of motivation, procrastination, or stress relief), then I would seriously encourage you to do your homework and follow these guidelines:

- Don't let just anyone put you under hypnosis.
- Make sure that the hypnotherapist is qualified.
- Make sure that the hypnotist is expertly trained.
- Ask if he or she has a background in mental health.
- Make sure that the hypnotist is thorough in his or her approach.
- As a rule of thumb, if it's cheap, then it's likely not the best help.

CHAPTER 14

Holiday Survival Guide

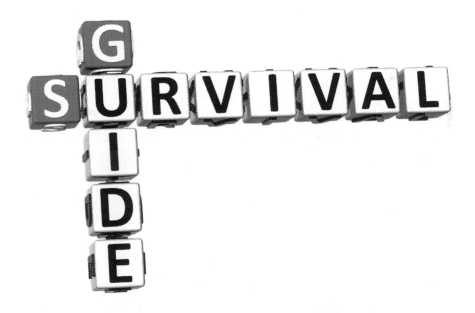

In this chapter, I'll provide helpful tips for not only surviving but also thriving during the holidays.

The holidays are upon us again! It's the time of the year when people try to get things wrapped up for work, start buying Christmas, Hanukkah, and Kwanzaa gifts, and start planning holiday activities with relatives and close friends.

All of this sounds positive, right? LOL. Well, it can also be *stressful*!

It's also the time of the year when finances can get tight, expenses may go through the roof, people get sick, people lose loved ones, workplace crises seem to rise, and many people get frustrated, anxious, stressed out, and even depressed. It's also the time of the year when all of this stress and anxiety may lead to colds and infections.

So, what can you do to enjoy the holidays while staving off all the unpleasant things I just mentioned? Well, you can do the most basic thing (your fallback) to make things go well: be *proactive*.

How? Here are some tips and tricks that will allow you to celebrate the holidays with joy, happiness, gratitude, empowerment, and abundance, while preventing frustration, stress, anxiety, depression, and even illness.

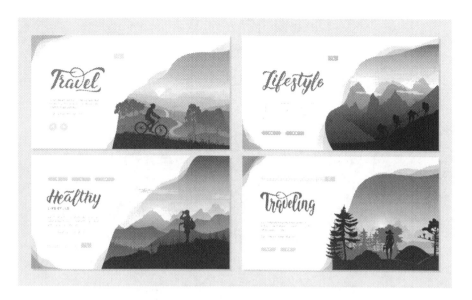

1. Create a plan and a schedule.

   Creating a schedule allows all the parts of your mind to be synchronized in terms of responsibilities and expectations. It gets all the voices in your brain on the same page. It helps you to organize the flow of your days, and it prevents little things from slipping off the list. You can use Post-it Notes and to-do lists to piece together your schedule, if that's easier.

   - Use a program (an app) on your phone, laptop, or desktop computer (such as Google Calendar or Apple's iCal) to build in reminders for your schedule of events. For instance, on iCal, you can schedule reminders one hour, two hours, one day, or two days (or any number of hours, days, weeks, or months) prior to the event. If you don't schedule in reminders, then you are much more likely to let smaller things fall through the cracks, especially when your schedule starts to get saturated.

- You can also attach documents, tickets, flyers, coupons, discount cards, and other things to the events in your schedule that will be needed when you arrive at your destination.
- Don't forget to schedule downtime and relaxation moments periodically so that you don't get overwhelmed by all the activity.

2. Create a realistic budget (but build in some degree of flexibility).

You are probably aware of this phenomenon, but many retailers make 80 percent to 90 percent of their profits between October and December (i.e., the last quarter of the year). While there are discount days and holiday specials, oftentimes the prices have already been hiked up (by hundreds of percentage points). So, create a budget for your holiday spending at the beginning of the year.

Yes, that's right! Create a budget and a list for your holiday shopping for the Christmas 2021 season in January of 2021. That's called real proactivity. You'll save hundreds (or even thousands) of dollars if you do this with all holidays, birthdays, celebrations, ceremonies, and other annual events. Buy all your 2021 gifts in January 2021, when the prices of everything (especially the big-ticket items) have been slashed. Beat the retailers at their own game!

Remember: proactivity beats reactivity every single day of the week. And it will prevent you from overspending during the holidays. It will also allow you to save money throughout the year (as prices slump, depending on the season), instead of paying the going market prices based on the season.

All of those warm sweaters that you're buying at 25 percent or 30 percent off right now (which have already been marked up 800 percent from cost) are 90 percent off during the summertime. So, buy them during the summertime, when they cost much less. And buy all your short-sleeved shirts during the wintertime. Doing this will also allow you to coast through the holidays while everyone else is scrambling to find that rare gift at the lowest price.

And you won't have to worry about all the really sought-after items disappearing on you.

3. Plan your diet (but build in cheats).

    Unfortunately, the holidays have become synonymous with overindulgence, sugary drinks and desserts, poor self-control, and weight gain. Part of the reason for this is all the holiday events and parties. However, you don't want to miss out on events just because you want to watch your calories. So, what do you do?

    Well, first you manage your diet and nutrition on a daily basis so that you can splurge when needed.

    Second, when you do splurge, do so in small increments.

    Basically, allow yourself to indulge in many different types of foods, but in smaller portions. So, instead of getting a huge wedge of that hot lasagna, get half a wedge. Also, eat smaller portions of dairy products such as cheeses, creamy dips and sauces.

    Third, when you're cooking, use spices to offset the need for fattening ingredients such as butter and heavy cream. For instance, use pesto instead of cheese. And when you do use cheese, use a less-fattening variety.

Another way to cut the calories is to consume your higher-calorie items during the earlier parts of the day (when you're most active). Moreover, consumer higher-calorie food during the parts of the day when you're most active.

Do take a multivitamin daily. And, don't take just any brand of multivitamin; take a high-quality one (e.g., GNC or Solgar).

Hypnosis is a really good tool for controlling urges and impulses to overindulge. Use all the tools at your disposal to manage what you eat.

The key is balance! Seek balance instead of deprivation; seek balance instead of overindulgence.

4. Remember, nothing is perfect (not even a diamond).

Many people strive to create the "perfect" holiday season.

My advice: Don't do it! Why? Because no matter what you do, it's not going to be perfect. There will be unexpected surprises, mishaps, challenges, obstacles, and distractions. Try to predict and manage for the most common, obvious, and/or detrimental of these, but don't lose heart if they happen no matter what you've done to prevent them.

That phrase about the best-laid plans comes to mind. Expect the unexpected. And when the unexpected happens, take a deep breath, relax, and move forward.

In general, trying to be perfect or to make things perfect doesn't work. In fact, aiming for perfection is a guarantee of failure. Don't aim for perfection. It's futile, and it will drive you, and the people around you, crazy.

5. Invite new people into your circle, and show gratitude to those around you.

   The holidays are an excellent occasion for inviting new people (and, hence, new energy and new ideas) into your circle. And those whom you invite into your circle are likely to be touched by, and appreciative of, your welcoming gesture(s).

   So, whom do you invite in? Invite an acquaintance or business associate with whom you've started to establish a good rapport. Why do this? Because it will enhance your circle of influence and will grow your personal brand. It will also help to inspire and create new connections among your friends and acquaintances. It will make you a "brand ambassador."

You see, regardless of whether you realize it or not, or notice it or not, you do have a brand and you are a brand. When people see, hear, and/or interact with you, they get a feeling, a sense, and an awareness of what you represent and stand for.

The more people you expose to your brand, the stronger it will become. Remember: *you* are your strongest advocate and your greatest asset.

6. Don't dare do it alone.

The best way to accomplish goals (especially large goals) is to break them up into more manageable pieces and then bring them altogether at the end.

Outsource things that you know that you don't like to do or don't do well. Enlist help from your friends, coworkers, and relatives. They will be honored that you trust them enough to help you.

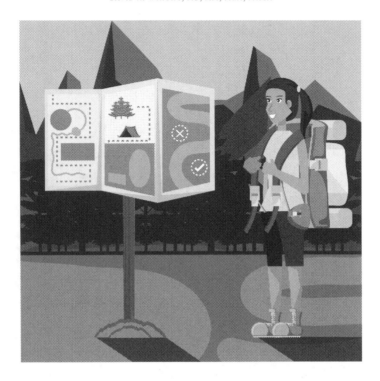

7. Schedule in relaxation, rejuvenation, and recuperation time.

Don't get burned out! Take the time to regroup, refresh, and reenergize.

If you're trying to do really important things while you're exhausted, the finished product will likely reflect that. So, know your limits and take a break whenever you reach those limits—even if it's just for five to ten minutes at a time. Use the time to meditate, nap, or do something menial. Doing something menial will relieve the parts of your brain that you've been overworking so they can take a much-deserved nap.

Or schedule a mental massage session.

8. Use music to tame your mood.

    Sounds and music are two of the most powerful means of shifting your mood and consciousness. *Hint:* That's why retailers (including clubs, pubs, lounges, and restaurants) use music and sounds: to drive sales.

    Check out the chapter on the power of sound and music in my book *Tomato Bisque for the Brain.*

    So, copy what the retailers have done. For instance, right now I'm really into Jens Buchert because he makes light, crisp minimalist music with repetitive rhythms that allow your mind to both relax and drift to new places. His music inspires you to dream, relax, and drift away, igniting parts of your brain that you don't normally use. It also helps you focus and concentrate while you work or study.

    Check out his music on Spotify, or on iTunes here: https://itunes.apple.com/us/artist/jens-buchert/15148392. The great thing about this service is that you can sample his music before you buy it.

9. Don't let anyone steal your peace, contentment, joy, bliss, or happiness.

   Most of us have a reason to be happy and joyous during the holidays. Some of these reasons might include family and friends, good health, and success. But not everyone has reasons to be happy.

   The holidays might be a challenging time for some individuals and/or families because the season may remind them of a loved one who has passed, a relationship that didn't work out, a career that hasn't panned out, or challenging financial times (e.g., a layoff or firing, inability to purchase gifts, another financial setback). If you encounter someone like this, acknowledge his or her experience, but don't allow the situation or the person to permanently dampen your positive mood for the day.

   If you desire to do so, say something kind or comforting. Or, if you so choose, just ignore the situation or the person.

But whatever you do, don't get sucked into the person's pattern, mood, or energy. And don't indulge his or her negativity. But do be empathetic, courteous, thoughtful, and kind.

How? By focusing on your core values—whatever those might be.

In general, the holidays are an excellent opportunity to recall, reset, and reorder your own values.

Values and beliefs drive our actions and our behaviors. However, occasionally we lose sight of one or more of our values. Use the season to get in better touch with your own values or to reevaluate some of them.

If you're struggling with your own values, then go to our website to read about our values-realignment service. It's *truly* life-changing. And definitely check out Dr. Adriana S. James's book *Values and the Evolution of Consciousness.* It's a must-read, especially if you find yourself in circumstances where you find a disconnect between your actions and behaviors and the values that you say that you have or desire to have. Dr. James is an expert in Neuro Linguistic Programming and Time Line Therapy ®. She is also an expert in the role of values on our behaviors, decisions and choices.

It's also good to explore your values if you have difficulty making decisions. Difficulties and dilemmas associated with decisions often occur when we perceive that one value collides with another value.

You can find Dr. James's book on Amazon.com. Dr. James is also the author of *Time Line Therapy Made Easy.* Time Line Therapy allows you to phenomenally change your outcomes and results in life. It's a core service that I recommend. You can read more about it under the Services tab on our website, or in our upcoming book *Alternative, Holistic, and Psychoanalytic Mental Health Approaches* (for those seeking therapies and life solutions without the use of psychotropic medications) (forthcoming).

10. Holiday Greetings!

For the past few decades, there seems to have been an ongoing war between saying "Merry Christmas" or "Happy Holidays." It probably won't end anytime soon. In my opinion, it's the thought (i.e., the sentiment) that counts more than the greeting itself.

But people get caught up in the details, and they get sensitive about things.

I'm not going to recommend what you should do. What I will do is tell you how I handle this situation.

I use the mirror technique, mirroring back the greeting that has been given to me. So, if someone says "Merry Christmas" or "Happy Holidays," then I'll say that back. I do the same with other greetings as well.

In my opinion, there are two things to remember when it comes to greetings (be they holiday or other greetings), regardless of your faith, religion, or belief system: (1) The thought/sentiment is what really matters. (2) Don't get bogged down in the details.

Details often separate us (because, if you boil anything down to minute details, there will be differences and distinctions), whereas core concepts (and, hence, values) often bring us all into alignment.

If you focus on values and core concepts (e.g., kindness, generosity, thoughtfulness, thankfulness, sharing, charity), you probably won't go wrong. And remember: You're *Never* going to please everyone, no matter what you say or do.

Try to spread positive vibes and energy, and leave the rest to God, the universe, energy, or whatever belief system to which you subscribe.

Of course, there's always "Seasons Greetings" and "Cheers!"

Cheers!

Merry Christmas, Happy Hanukkah, Splendid Kwanzaa, Happy Holidays, and Seasons Greetings!

CHAPTER 15

General Health and Mental Health Nuggets

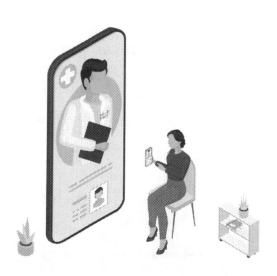

These are the platinum, gold, silver, and bronze nuggets for general health, wellness, diet, weight loss, weight management, and mental health.

Welcome to the *best* superlist of general health, wellness, diet, nutrition, weight loss, weight management, mental health, lifestyle, abundance, empowerment, prosperity, and success nuggets that you've ever come across—all in one place, where you can come back to it over and over again quickly in order to get yourself back on course if and when you stray from your desired pathway.

1. You have to have a vision, a mission, goals, plans, and strategies.

2. You must have a purpose, a passion, a pursuit, and a plan.

3. Work with your healthcare providers, especially your primary care physician (PCP).

4. Work with your therapist, counselor, coach, and/or psychiatrist.

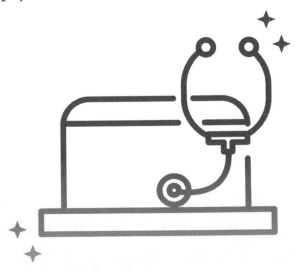

5. Ask your medicine prescribers to help you by choosing medications that are weight neutral or weight negative. For instance, you might request an SSRI (such as Prozac or Trintellix) that can be taken in the morning, versus a TCA (such as Elavil) that is taken at night, if you have depression or insomnia.

6. Realize that antihistamines, especially older ones such as Benadryl and hydroxyzine, can cause you to gain weight. Instead of using those, try allergy medicines that have fewer cholinergic side effects such as Claritin, Zyrtec, Xyzal, and Allegra.

7. Lower your stress and anxiety using exercise, meditation, yoga, and other activities.

8. Realize that inflammatory states may also lead to weight gain or weight maintenance.

9. Use your diet to help control and reduce symptoms of acid reflux and GERD, especially if they are new. Believe it or not, your body may be trying to tell you something, such as to eat dinner earlier and consume smaller meals.

10. Realize that many drugs used to treat acid reflux and GERD often make it worse over time if you

fail to address the underlying root causes of these conditions.

11. Realize that some diabetes drugs may cause weight gain. Ask your PCP for alternatives that are either weight neutral or weight negative.

12. Many psychiatric/psychotropic drugs used to treat psychiatric conditions such as bipolar disorder and schizophrenia can cause weight gain. Know this ahead of time, and plan for it by changing your dietary and activity habits— which will serendipitously help with your mental health symptoms too.

13. Realize that your weight, your health-related symptoms, and other challenges you experience are simply symptoms of a greater root cause. While you work on the symptoms, get to the root causes and work on those.

14. Realize that if you take or use stimulants (such as Vyvanse, Adderall, Ritalin [God forbid], nicotine, or caffeine), when you quit taking or using them, your metabolism will slow down and you will have to deal with two related circumstances that will cause your weight to increase very quickly if you don't pay close attention: (1) an increased appetite and (2) a slower metabolism. Given this

fact, if you are planning to come off one or more of these substances, you should get help from a professional.

15. In general, except for things like water, there is an inverse relationship between nutritional value and shelf life. The longer something can stay on the shelf (or in your pantry) and still be healthily consumed, the less nutritious it is for you. That's because the food producers have to remove nutrients that can't sit on the shelves from the products and put in additives that extend the life of any nutrients that are left that can take living on the shelves (or in your pantry, LOL). That's why so many people eat only farm-to-table organic foods. By the way, many of these additives can cause allergies and inflammation. So, while you don't have to remove shelf items from your diet, be sure to limit your exposure. One exception might be some items that are able to stay on the shelves because they are preserved in oils. Even then, it's still better to have fresh items.

16. Perhaps this should be rather obvious, but it's not healthy to eat live animals or reptiles. Please stay away from that appetizing live mouse or bat. It's probably not good for you, and it's a great way to

pass viruses and diseases from another species to ours. That should be obvious, but clearly, in the midst of this COVID-19 pandemic, it isn't.

17. Keep it simple, be creative, take safe risks, and seek balance and compromise.

18. Never clear your plate while you're trying to lose weight.

19. Many people assume that they are not at higher risk for getting very ill from COVID-19 because they aren't chronically ill and aren't being treated with multiple medications. They are wrong. Here are some hidden risk factors for morbidity and mortality arising from COVID-19:

a. Being overweight
b. Being obese
c. Being morbidly obese
d. Having metabolic syndrome (diabetes, hypertension, obesity, etc.)
e. Having chronic bronchitis, emphysema, or COPD (chronic obstructive pulmonary disease)
f. Smoking cigarettes
g. Smoking Black & Milds
h. Smoking cigars
i. Smoking marijuana

j. Vaping

k. Having obstructive sleep apnea (OSA)

20. If you're having sleep problems, you have to fix them. My first self-improvement, self-empowerment, self-determination, and self-development book, *Sweet Potato Pie for the Spirit, Soul, and Psyche*, dedicates an entire chapter to explaining the process of sleep and provides you with a host of methods to fix your sleep dilemmas, naturally and holistically.

CHAPTER 16

Putting It All Together

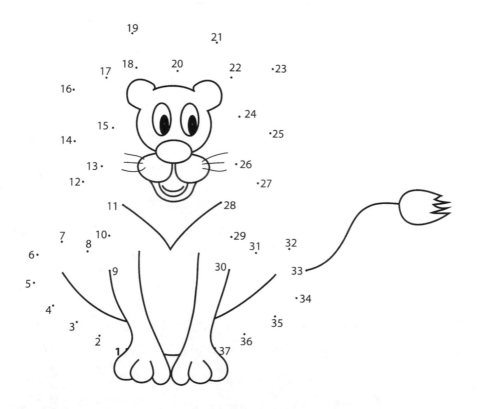

In a very real sense, this was the easiest chapter to write because we've covered all the basics in prior chapters. But it's always helpful to weave it all together and tie up loose ends. That leads me to basic concepts to keep in mind:

1. Use technology to help you, not to enslave you.

2. Use others to help motivate you and keep you motivated.

3. Choose things that you like and enjoy.

4. Choose behaviors over calories. If you feel that you have to choose, then choose the best behavior over the lower calorie count. For instance, eating a balanced meal with vegetables, protein, and fiber is more important than eating rice cakes just because they are lower in calories. It really isn't just about the calories.

5. Your beverage behaviors are every bit as important as your food behaviors, especially considering the fact that your body is 66 percent water (i.e., liquid).

6. Keep in mind that in order to maintain your desired weight goals, they *must* be *sustainable*. In other words, you have to be able to live with them. So, find balances and compromises that work for and with you.

7. Have *realistic* body weight and shape goals. The biggest enemy of a successful weight management and lifestyle program is unrealistic expectations.

8. Keep it lighthearted, simple, and fun. If you make it complicated or super-duper stringent, and/or if you approach it in an anal-retentive way, then you're going to gain weight because of the additional stress, anxiety, anticipation, and expectations.

9. Start with a physician, lifestyle, or mental health coach who understands medicine, nutrition, and psychology.

10. Be willing to fail. Most people fail multiple times before they are successful, regardless of whether we're talking about quitting smoking or changing diet and lifestyle choices and decisions. And most people either don't try in the first place or give up just before a turning point because they fear failing. Be the *exception*. Be willing and ready to fail as many times as it takes in order to reach your goals and ambitions because it's that important to you, and because you aren't willing to give up without a fight (or two, or three, or four, or five).

CHAPTER 17

Conclusions

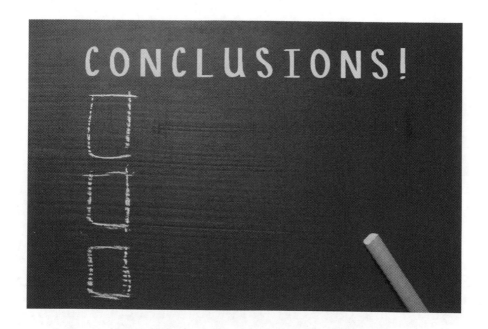

The vast majority of diet plans and approaches fail because they expect the individual to make too many primary changes at once. In essence, they expect the person to change overnight—which rarely happens anywhere in nature (including within humanity). Plans, goals, and objectives tend to fail when they require too many steps too quickly. I base this opinion on the simplicity principle, which states that the simpler something is to set up and begin, the more likely one is to consistently continue (i.e., perpetuate) it. The reverse of that is the complexity principle, which states that the more complicated something is to set up, begin, and perpetuate, the more likely one is to abruptly discontinue (i.e., abandon) it.

Lifestyle choices and changes are no different from any other choices, decisions, or changes. You're much more likely to be successful if you create and continue one new lifestyle habit each week for a certain amount of time. Now all that you have to do is choose which lifestyle choices that you'd like to add (or remove) each week for fifty-four weeks—or in this case, only twelve weeks (i.e., three months). I always recommend beginning with the basics (i.e., the building blocks). Start with what you do when you first awaken in the morning, and go from there until you reach the end of the day—until you have the week mapped out. Then you can look at the weekend and move on from there to the details that are individualistic in nature.

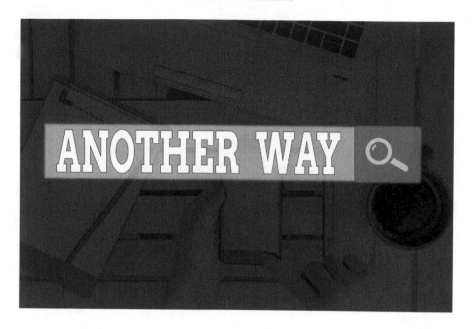

The Nutrient Diet is a completely new, bold, different, psychological approach to diet, health, wellness, and weight-management habits. It's a lifestyle book for general and mental health based on sound psychological principles. *The Nutrient Diet* is 50 percent about diet and nutrition and 50 percent about cognitive and behavioral psychological strategies for eating behaviors, dieting, impulse control, and habit formation. It's the first book of its kind to take a cognitive behavioral (i.e., psychological) approach to diet, nutrition, health, wellness, and lifestyle management. It truly is a trendsetter in the diet, health, wellness, medicine, nutrition, and lifestyle fields. Not only does *The Nutrient Diet* show and explain what you need to eat, but it also explains *how* you should eat it—based on sound, tested scientific data and psychological principles. And it does this in a way that allows you to make lifestyle changes easily, naturally, and progressively so that you don't get overwhelmed.

I've also used the principles, techniques, and methods of habit formation to help my clients who are seeking abundance, empowerment, courage, confidence, prosperity, and direction to successfully change careers, double their incomes, move past procrastination and stagnation, lose substantial amounts of weight, and re-create happiness and joy in their lives. *The Nutrient Diet* shows you how to use your thoughts, feelings, moods, actions, reactions, habits, and belief systems so they become allies in your weight-management, diet, and lifestyle goals. Together, these tools, methods, resources, strategies, and approaches positively change the trajectory of your life—while simultaneously adding joy, happiness, and fulfillment to it. The keys to diet, weight management, and impulse control are habit and ritual creation, formation, and sustainment. *The Nutrient Diet* helps you build a daily self-care regimen that works for you. It helps you to care for your mind and body in a way that empowers you daily, while preventing frustration, stagnation, and exhaustion. And if you use it with my other books (which have tools to help support a mindset that encompasses healthy habits, choices, and rituals), which introduce and draw upon alternative mental health and wellness techniques such as hypnosis, hypnotherapy, mindfulness, mind-setting, NLP (neurolinguistic programming), and Time Line Therapy, then you will have a foolproof tool for a healthier, happier lifestyle and greater well-being. Your dietary and wellness history has definitely helped to shape who and what you are today, but the negative aspects of your history don't have to define who you will be in the future. You, and you alone, get to *define*, *develop*, and *defend* your *desires* and your *destiny*. You've started the journey to determine, develop, and define your desires and your destiny by using the techniques, methods, and resources introduced here. Along the way you might slip. You might even fall. But if you continue to employ the techniques and methods that you've learned here, you will never, ever stay on the ground. You've become *tougher*! You've become *stronger*! You've become a *fighter*! And that's what it takes to win the battle for your *destiny*! It truly is all about those little steps that you take on a daily basis. I like to call them habits.

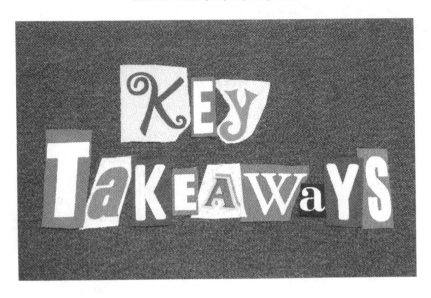

Finally, move forward confidently in the knowledge that most people fail multiple times before they succeed at something, especially something that is habitual or important. Did you succeed the very first time you attempted to walk? Probably not. Did you succeed the very first time you attempted to ride a bike? Probably not. Did you succeed the very first time you attempted to write a letter of the alphabet? Probably not. Did you succeed the very first day of your very first job? Probably not. *The Nutrient Diet* is not about being perfect. Instead, it's about learning an approach to habit creation, formation, and maintenance so that you don't have try to be perfect. At its essence, it presents a human (i.e., cognitive behavioral) approach to lifestyle management. And it gives you permission to be imperfect—a characteristic that other diet and lifestyle plans fail to provide.

REFERENCES

"6 Reasons Tempeh Should Be Part of a Healthy Diet." May 22, 2017. Ecowatch. https://www.ecowatch.com/tempeh-healthy-diet-2418024546.html.

Abbasi, J. "Interest in the Ketogenic Diet Grows for Weight Loss and Type 2 Diabetes." *Journal of the American Medical Association* 319, no. 3 (2018): 215–17.

Acocella, J. "A Few Too Many: Is There Hope for the Hung Over?" *New Yorker*, May 26, 2008. http://www.newyorker.com/magazine/2008/05/26/a-few-too-many.

Arnarson, A. "7 Evidence-Based Ways to Prevent Hangovers," Healthline, June 15, 2017. http://www.healthline.com/nutrition/7-ways-to-prevent-a-hangover.

Aubrey, Allison. "Want to Avoid a Hangover? Science Has Got You Covered." NPR, December 31, 2015. http://www.npr.org/sections/thesalt/2015/12/31/461594898/want-to-avoid-a-hangover-science-has-got-you-covered.

Barclay, A. W., P. Petocz, J. McMillan-Price, et al. "Glycemic Index, Glycemic Load, and Chronic Disease Risk—a Meta-Analysis of Observational Studies." *American Journal of Clinical Nutrition* 87, no. 3 (2008): 627–37. https://doi.org/10.1093/ajcn/87.3.627. Retrieved from https://www.ncbi.nlm.nih.gov/pubmed/18326601.

Bharanidharan, Sadhana. "Is Drinking Milk Good for You? 3 Pros and Cons," Medical Daily, August 20, 2018. https://www.medicaldaily.com/ drinking-milk-good-you-3-pros-and-cons-426975.

Bifari F, Ruocco C, Decimo I, Fumagalli G, Valerio A, Nisoli E. Amino acid supplements and metabolic health: a potential interplay between intestinal microbiota and systems control. Genes Nutr. 2017;12:27. Published 2017 Oct 4. doi:10.1186/ s12263-017-0582-2

Bjarnadottir, MS, RDN. How Drinking More Water Can Help You Lose Weight. Healthline, 2017. Retrieved from https://www.healthline. com/nutrition/drinking-water-helps-with-weight-loss.

Boden, G., K. Sargrad, C. Homko, M. Mozzoli, and T. P. Stein. "Effect of a Low-Carbohydrate Diet on Appetite, Blood Glucose Levels, and Insulin Resistance in Obese Patients with Type 2 Diabetes." *Annals of Internal Medicine* 142, no. 6 (2005): 403–11. https://doi.org/10.7326/0003-4819-142-6-200503150- 00006. Retrieved from https://www.ncbi.nlm.nih.gov/ pubmed/15767618.

Boschmann M, Steiniger J, Hille U, et al. Water-induced thermogenesis. J Clin Endocrinol Metab. 2003;88(12):6015-6019. doi:10.1210/ jc.2003-030780. Retrieved from https://www.ncbi.nlm.nih. gov/pubmed/14671205

Børsheim E, Bui QU, Tissier S, Kobayashi H, Ferrando AA, Wolfe RR. Effect of amino acid supplementation on muscle mass, strength and physical function in elderly. Clin Nutr. 2008;27(2):189-195. doi:10.1016/j.clnu.2008.01.001

Bough, K. J., and J. M. Rho. "Anticonvulsant Mechanisms of the Ketogenic Diet." *Epilepsia* 48 (2007): 43–58. https://doi. org/10.1111/j.1528-1167.2007.00915.x.

Brehm, B. J., R. J. Seeley, S. R. Daniels, and D. A. D'Alessio. "A Randomized Trial Comparing a Very Low Carbohydrate Diet and a Calorie-Restricted Low Fat Diet on Body Weight and Cardiovascular Risk Factors in Healthy Women." *Journal of Clinical Endocrinology and Metabolism* 88, no. 4 (2003): 1617–23. https://doi.org/10.1210/jc.2002-021480. Retrieved from https://www.ncbi.nlm.nih.gov/pubmed/12679447.

Brondo, Sammi. "Sammi's Nutrition Tips: The Complete Guide to Snacking." https://www.sammibrondo.com/blog/guide-to-snacking.

Bueno, N., I. De Melo, S. De Oliveira, and T. Da Rocha Ataide. "Very-Low-Carbohydrate Ketogenic Diet v. Low-Fat Diet for Long-Term Weight Loss: A Meta-Analysis of Randomised Controlled Trials." *British Journal of Nutrition* 110, no. 7 (2013): 1178–87.

Centr Team. "Snacking Guidelines." https://centr.com/article/show/5157/cen-snacking-guidelines.

Coello, K., M. Vinberg, F. K. Knop, et al. "Metabolic Profile in Patients with Newly Diagnosed Bipolar Disorder and Their Unaffected First-Degree Relatives." *International Journal of Bipolar Disorder* (April 2, 2019). https://doi.org/10.1186/s40345-019-0142-3.

Collins, N. "Hangover Cures: What Does the Science Say?" *Telegraph*, October 10, 2013. http://www.telegraph.co.uk/news/health/news/10366146/Hangover-cures-what-does-the-science-say.html.

Cummings NE, Williams EM, Kasza I, et al. Restoration of metabolic health by decreased consumption of branched-chain amino acids. J Physiol. 2018;596(4):623-645. doi:10.1113/JP275075

Cunnane, S. C., and M. A. Crawford. "Survival of the Fattest: Fat Babies Were the Key to Evolution of the Large Human Brain." *Comparative Biochemistry and Physiology Part A, Molecular & Integrative Physiology* 136, no. 1 (2003): 17–26. https://doi.

org/10.1016/s1095-6433(03)00048-5. Retrieved from https://www.ncbi.nlm.nih.gov/pubmed/14527626.

Davy BM, Dennis EA, Dengo AL, Wilson KL, Davy KP. Water consumption reduces energy intake at a breakfast meal in obese older adults. J Am Diet Assoc. 2008;108(7):1236-1239. doi:10.1016/j.jada.2008.04.013. Retrieved from https://www.ncbi.nlm.nih.gov/pubmed/18589036

Dehghan, M., A. Mente, X. Zhang, et al. "Associations of Fats and Carbohydrate Intake with Cardiovascular Disease and Mortality in 18 Countries from Five Continents (PURE): A Prospective Cohort Study." *Lancet* (August 28, 2017). https://doi.org/10.1016/S0140-6736(17)32252-3.

Dillon EL, Sheffield-Moore M, Paddon-Jones D, Gilkison C, Sanford AP, Casperson SL, Jiang J, Chinkes DL, Urban RJ. Amino acid supplementation increases lean body mass, basal muscle protein synthesis, and insulin-like growth factor-I expression in older women. J Clin Endocrinol Metab. 2009 May;94(5):1630-7. doi: 10.1210/jc.2008-1564. Epub 2009 Feb 10. PMID: 19208731; PMCID: PMC2684480.

"The Dish on Dairy: Are Dairy Foods Healthy, or Is It Best to Reduce or Even Avoid Them in Your Diet?" *Harvard Men's Health Watch*, February 2019. https://www.health.harvard.edu/staying-healthy/the-dish-on-dairy.

Dupuis, N., N. Curatolo, J. F. Benoist, and S. Auvin. "Ketogenic Diet Exhibits Anti-Inflammatory Properties." *Epilepsia* 56 (2015): e95–e98.

Ebbeling, C. B., J. F. Swain, H. A. Feldman, W. W. Wong, D. L. Hachey, E. Garcia-Lago, and D. S. Ludwig. "Effects of Dietary Composition on Energy Expenditure during Weight-Loss Maintenance." *Journal of the American Medical Association* 307, no. 24 (2012): 2627–34. https://doi.org/10.1001/jama.2012.6607.

Ede, Georgia. "Low-Carbohydrate Diet Superior to Antipsychotic Medications: Two Remarkable Personal Stories as Told by Their Harvard Psychiatrist." *Psychology Today*, September 29, 2017.

"Effects of Alcohol Use. Understand the Long-Term and Short-Term Effects of Alcohol before Drinking." Caron. https://www.caron.org/understanding-addiction/alcoholism/effects-of-alcohol.

English KL, Paddon-Jones D. Protecting muscle mass and function in older adults during bed rest. Curr Opin Clin Nutr Metab Care. 2010;13(1):34-39. doi:10.1097/MCO.0b013e328333aa66

Fantozzi, J. "Watch What Alcohol Does to Your Body: It's Not Pretty." The Daily Meal, July 10, 2015. https://www.thedailymeal.com/news/drink/watch-what-alcohol-does-your-body-it-s-not-pretty/071015.

Feinman, R. D., and M. Makowske. "Metabolic Syndrome and Low-Carbohydrate Ketogenic Diets in the Medical School Biochemistry Curriculum." *Metabolic Syndrome and Related Disorders* 1, no. 3 (2003): 189–97. https://doi.org/10.1089/154041903322716660. Retrieved from https://www.ncbi.nlm.nih.gov/pubmed/18370662.

Felson, Sabrina. "Drinking Water Quality: What You Need to Know." WebMD, October 23, 2018. https://www.webmd.com/women/safe-drinking-water.

Fine, E. J., C. J. Segal-Isaacson, R. D. Feinman, et al. "Targeting Insulin Inhibition as a Metabolic Therapy in Advanced Cancer: A Pilot Safety and Feasibility Dietary Trial in 10 Patients." *Nutrition* 28, no. 10 (2012): 1028–35. https://doi.org/10.1016/j.nut.2012.05.001. Retrieved from https://www.ncbi.nlm.nih.gov/pubmed/22840388/.

Frakti. "The Effects of Alcohol on Your Body." DrugAbuse.com. http://drugabuse.com/featured/the-effects-of-alcohol-on-the-body/.

Freeman, J. M., E. P. G. Vining, E. H. Kossoff, et al. "A Blinded, Crossover Study of the Ketogenic Diet." *Epilepsia* 50 (2009): 322–25.

Freeman, J. M., E. P. Vining, D. J. Pillas, P. L. Pyzik, J. C. Casey, and L. M. Kelly. "The Efficacy of the Ketogenic Diet—1998: A Prospective Evaluation of Intervention in 150 Children." *Pediatrics* 102, no. 6 (1998): 1358–63. https://doi.org/10.1542/peds.102.6.1358. Retrieved from https://www.ncbi.nlm.nih.gov/pubmed/9832569.

Fujita S, Volpi E. Amino acids and muscle loss with aging. J Nutr. 2006;136(1 Suppl):277S-80S. doi:10.1093/jn/136.1.277S

Fukao, T., G. D. Lopaschuk, and G. A. Mitchell. "Pathways and Control of Ketone Body Metabolism: On the Fringe of Lipid Biochemistry." *Prostaglandins, Leukotrines, & Essential Fatty Acids* 70, no. 3 (2004): 243–51. https://doi.org/10.1016/j.plefa.2003.11.001. Retrieved from https://www.ncbi.nlm.nih.gov/pubmed/14769483.

"The Functions of Carbohydrates in the Body." EUFIC, January 14, 2020. https://www.eufic.org/en/whats-in-food/article/the-basics-carbohydrates.

Furth, S. L., J. C. Casey, P. L. Pyzik, et al. "Risk Factors for Urolithiasis in Children on the Ketogenic Diet." *Pediatric Nephrology* 15, no. 1–2 (2000): 125–28. https://doi.org/10.1007/s004670000443. Retrieved from https://www.ncbi.nlm.nih.gov/pubmed/11095028.

Galvan E, Arentson-Lantz E, Lamon S, Paddon-Jones D. Protecting Skeletal Muscle with Protein and Amino Acid during Periods of Disuse. Nutrients. 2016;8(7):404. Published 2016 Jul 1. doi:10.3390/nu8070404

Gibson, A. A., R. V. Seimon, C. M. Lee, et al. "Do Ketogenic Diets Really Suppress Appetite? A Systematic Review and Meta-Analysis." *Obesity Reviews* 16, no. 1 (2015): 64–76. https://doi.

org/10.1111/obr.12230. Retrieved from https://www.ncbi.nlm.nih.gov/pubmed/25402637.

Gibson EL, Vargas K, Hogan E, et al. Effects of acute treatment with a tryptophan-rich protein hydrolysate on plasma amino acids, mood and emotional functioning in older women. Psychopharmacology (Berl). 2014;231(24):4595-4610. doi:10.1007/s00213-014-3609-z

Gilbert-Jaramillo, J., D. Vargas-Pico, T. Espinosa-Mendoza, S. Falk, K. Llanos-Fernández, J. Guerrero-Haro, C. Orellana-Román, C. Poveda-Loor, J. Valdevila-Figueira, and C. M. Palmer. "The Effects of the Ketogenic Diet on psychiatric Symptomatology, Weight, and Metabolic Dysfunction in Schizophrenia Patients." *Clinical Nutrition and Metabolism* 1, no. 1 (July 31, 2018): 1–5. https://doi.org/10.15761/CNM.100010.

Goodman, Brenda. "Rethinking Milk: Science Takes On the Dairy Dilemma." WebMD. https://www.webmd.com/diet/news/20200214/rethinking-mik-science-takes-on-the-dairy-dilemma.

Gosmanov, A. R., E. O. Gosmanova, and E. Dillard-Cannon. "Management of Adult Diabetic Ketoacidosis," *Diabetes, Metabolic Syndrome, and Obesity* 7 (June 30, 2014): 255–64. https://doi.org/10.2147/DMSO.S50516. Retrieved from https://www.ncbi.nlm.nih.gov/pubmed/25061324/.

Gunnars, Kris. "How Much Water Should You Drink Per Day?" Healthline, June 20, 2018. https://www.healthline.com/nutrition/how-much-water-should-you-drink-per-day.

Harkinson, Josh. "The Scary New Science that Shows Milk Is Bad for You: Evidence Suggests Dairy Doesn't Do a Body Good—So Why Does the Government Still Push Three Servings a Day?" *Mother Jones*, November–December 2015. https://www.motherjones.com/environment/2015/11/dairy-industry-milk-federal-dietary-guidelines/.

Hasselbalch, S. G., G. M. Knudsen, J. Jakobsen, L. P. Hageman, S. Holm, and O. B. Paulson. "Brain Metabolism during Short-Term Starvation in Humans." *Journal of Cerebral Blood Flow and Metabolism* 14, no. 1 (1994): 125–31. https://doi.org/10.1038/jcbfm.1994.17. Retrieved from https://www.ncbi.nlm.nih.gov/pubmed/8263048/.

"Healthy Snacking." Heart.org. https://www.heart.org/en/healthy-living/healthy-eating/add-color/healthy-snacking.

Helms ER, Aragon AA, Fitschen PJ. Evidence-based recommendations for natural bodybuilding contest preparation: nutrition and supplementation. J Int Soc Sports Nutr. 2014;11:20. Published 2014 May 12. doi:10.1186/1550-2783-11-20

Henderson, S. T., J. L. Vogel, L. J, Barr, F. Garvin, J. J. Jones, and L. C. Costantini. "Study of the Ketogenic Agent AC-1202 in Mild to Moderate Alzheimer's Disease: A Randomized, Double-Blind, Placebo-Controlled, Multicenter Trial." *Nutrition & Metabolism* (London) 6 (August 10, 2009): 31. https://doi.org/10.1186/1743-7075-6-31. Retrieved from https://www.ncbi.nlm.nih.gov/pubmed/19664276/.

Holeček M. Branched-chain amino acids in health and disease: metabolism, alterations in blood plasma, and as supplements. Nutr Metab (Lond). 2018;15:33. Published 2018 May 3. doi:10.1186/s12986-018-0271-1

Hopper, J. W., Z. Su, A. R. Looby, E. T. Ryan, D. M. Penetar, C. M. Palmer, and S. E. Lukas. "Incidence and Patterns of Polydrug Use and Craving for Ecstasy in Regular Ecstasy Users: An Ecological Momentary Assessment Study." *Drug and Alcohol Dependency* 85, no. 3 (December 1, 2006): 221–35. https://doi.org/10.1016/j.drugalcdep.2006.04.012.

Hrefna, Palsdottir. "What Is Ketosis, and Is It Healthy?" Healthline, June 3, 2017. https://www.healthline.com/nutrition/what-is-ketosis.https://snacknation.com/blog/guide/healthy-snacks/.

Hu C, Li F, Duan Y, Yin Y, Kong X. Dietary Supplementation With Leucine or in Combination With Arginine Decreases Body Fat Weight and Alters Gut Microbiota Composition in Finishing Pigs. Front Microbiol. 2019;10:1767. Published 2019 Aug 13. doi:10.3389/fmicb.2019.01767

Iftikhar, Noreen. "Pros and Cons of Drinking Cow's Milk," Healthline, May 11, 2020.

Jenkins TA, Nguyen JC, Polglaze KE, Bertrand PP. Influence of Tryptophan and Serotonin on Mood and Cognition with a Possible Role of the Gut-Brain Axis. Nutrients. 2016;8(1):56. Published 2016 Jan 20. doi:10.3390/nu8010056

Kang, H. C., Y. J. Kim, D. W. Kim, and H. D. Kim. "Efficacy and Safety of the Ketogenic Diet for Intractable Childhood Epilepsy: Korean Multicentric Experience." *Epilepsia* 46, no. 2 (2005): 272–79. https://doi.org/10.1111/j.0013-9580.2005.48504.x. Retrieved from https://www.ncbi.nlm.nih.gov/pubmed/15679508.

Khan Academy. "Introduction to Proteins and Amino Acids." https://www.khanacademy.org/science/biology/macromolecules/proteins-and-amino-acids/a/introduction-to-proteins-and-amino-acids.

Kielb, S., H. P. Koo, D. A. Bloom, and G. I. Faerber. "Nephrolithiasis Associated with the Ketogenic Diet." *Journal of Urology* 164, no. 2 (200): 464–66. https://www.ncbi.nlm.nih.gov/pubmed/10893623.

"Know Your Limits." Know … the Effects of Alcohol. http://www.knowyourlimits.info/know%E2%80%A6-effects-alcohol.

Koenig, Debbie. "Can You Eat to Beat Depression?" WebMD, December 2, 2019.

Koren, Talia. "Meal Prep Snacks: The Best Snacks to Take to Work or School." Work Week Lunch,

February 18, 2020. https://workweeklunch.com/ultimate-guide-healthy-snacking/.

Kraeuter, A. K., H. Loxton, B. C. Lima, D. Rudd, and Z. Sarnyai. "Ketogenic Diet Reverses Behavioral Abnormalities in an Acute NMDA Receptor Hypofunction Model of Schizophrenia." *Schizophrenia Research* 169 (2015): 491–93.

Kraft and Westman. "Schizophrenia, Gluten, and Low-Carbohydrate, Ketogenic Diets: A Case Report and Review of the Literature." *Nutrition & Metabolism* 6 (2009): 10.

Kuzma, C. "This is Your Body on Booze." *Men's Health*, October 12, 2015. http://www.menshealth.com/health/your-body-on-booze

LaManna, J. C., N. Salem, M. Puchowicz, et al. "Ketones Suppress Brain Glucose Consumption." *Advances in Experimental Medicine and Biology* 645 (2009): 301–6. https://doi.org/10.1007/978-0-387-85998-9_45. Retrieved from https://www.ncbi.nlm.nih.gov/pubmed/19227486/.

Levy, R. G., P. N. Cooper, and P. Giri. "Ketogenic Diet and Other Dietary Treatments for Epilepsy." *Cochrane Database of Systematic Reviews* 3 (March 14, 2012): CD001903. https://doi.org/10.1002/14651858.CD001903.pub2. Retrieved from https://www.ncbi.nlm.nih.gov/pubmed/22419282.

Li, H. F., Y. Zou, and G. Ding. "Therapeutic Success of the Ketogenic Diet as a Treatment Option for Epilepsy: A Meta-Analysis." *Iranian Journal of Pediatrics* 23, no. 6 (2013): 613–20. https://www.ncbi.nlm.nih.gov/pubmed/24910737.

Licata, S. C., D. M. Penetar, C. Ravichandran, J. Rodolico, C. Palmer, J. Berko, T. Geaghan, A. Looby, E. Peters, E. Ryan, P. F. Renshaw, and S. E. Lukas. "Effects of Daily Treatment with Citicoline: A Double-Blind, Placebo-Controlled Study in Cocaine-Dependent Volunteers." *Journal of Addiction*

Medicine 5, no. 1 (March 2011): 57–64. https://doi.org/10.1097/ ADM.0b013e3181d80c93.

Liu, S., W. C. Willett, M. J. Stampfer, et al. "A Prospective Study of Dietary Glycemic Load, Carbohydrate Intake, and Risk of Coronary Heart Disease in US Women." *American Journal of Clinical Nutrition* 71, no. 6 (2000): 1455–61. https://doi. org/10.1093/ajcn/71.6.1455. Retrieved from https://pubmed. ncbi.nlm.nih.gov/10837285/.

Love, Shayla. "The Sugar High Might Be a Myth." *Vice*, April 12, 2019. https://www.vice.com/en/article/gy4pg3/ the-sugar-high-might-be-a-myth.

Ludwig, David. "Time to Question Everything You Know about Milk." February 12 (n.y.). Elemental Medium. https:// elemental.medium.com/time-to-question-everything-you-know-about-milk-12c08b13e98a.

Lukas, S. E., D. Penetar, Z. Su, T. Geaghan, M. Maywalt, M. Tracy, J. Rodolico, C. Palmer, Z. Ma, and D. Y. Lee. "A Standardized Kudzu Extract (NPI-031) Reduces Alcohol Consumption in Nontreatment-Seeking Male Heavy Drinkers." *Psychopharmacology* (Berlin) 226, no. 1 (March 2013): 65–73. https://doi.org/10.1007/s00213-012-2884-9.

Lukas, S. E., S. B. Lowen, K. P. Lindsey, N. Conn, W. Tartarini, J. Rodolico, G. Mallya, C. Palmer, and D. M. Penetar. "Extended-Release Naltrexone (XR-NTX) Attenuates Brain Responses to Alcohol Cues in Alcohol-Dependent Volunteers: A Bold FMRI Study." *Neuroimage* 78 (September 2013): 176–85. https://doi.org/10.1016/j.neuroimage.2013.03.055.

Lukas, S.E., D. Penetar, J. Berk, L. Vicens, C. Palmer, G. Mallya, E. A. Macklin, and D. Y. Lee. "An Extract of the Chinese Herbal Root Kudzu Reduces Alcohol Drinking by Heavy Drinkers in a Naturalistic Setting." *Alcoholism: Clinical and*

Experimental Research 29, no. 5 (May 2005): 756–62. https://doi.org/10.1097/01.alc.0000163499.64347.92.

Lung Health. "21 Foods that Trigger Mucus Production (and 21 Foods that Reduce It)." Lung Institute, December 26, 2017. https://lunginstitute.com/blog/21-foods-trigger-mucus-production-21-foods-reduce/.

Luo, E. K. "The Effects of Alcohol on Your Body," Healthline, June 9, 2017. http://www.healthline.com/health/alcohol/effects-on-body.

Magee, A. "What Alcohol Does to Your Body after the Age of 40." *Telegraph*, December 14, 2015. http://www.telegraph.co.uk/health-fitness/body/what-alcohol-does-to-your-body-after-the-age-of-40/.

Mana Medical Associates. "Dairy Products Pros and Cons." https://www.mana.md/dairy-products-pros-and-cons/.

Marcin, Ashley. "How Much Water You Need to Drink." Healthline, November 2, 2018. https://www.healthline.com/health/how-much-water-should-I-drink.

———. "Brown Fat: What You Should Know." Healthline, January 22, 2018. https://www.healthline.com/health/brown-fat#1.

Martin, K., C. F. Jackson, R. G. Levy, and P. N. Cooper. "Ketogenic Diet and Other Dietary Treatments for Epilepsy." *Cochrane Database of Systematic Reviews* 2 (2016): CD001903. https://doi.org/10.1002/14651858.CD001903.pub3.

McClernon, F. J., W. S. Yancy Jr., J. A. Eberstein, R. C. Atkins, and E. C. Westman. "The Effects of a Low-Carbohydrate Ketogenic Diet and a Low-Fat Diet on Mood, Hunger, and Other Self-Reported Symptoms." *Obesity* (Silver Spring) 15, no. 1 (2007): 182–87. https://doi.org/10.1038/oby.2007.516. Retrieved from https://www.ncbi.nlm.nih.gov/pubmed/17228046.

McGuire, L. C., A. M. Cruickshank, and P. T. Munro. "Alcoholic Ketoacidosis." *Emergency Medicine Journal* 23, no. 6 (2006): 417–20. https://doi.org/10.1136/emj.2004.017590. Retrieved from https://www.ncbi.nlm.nih.gov/pubmed/16714496.

Medlin, Sophie. "Do Humans Need Dairy? Here's the Science." The Conversation, December 14, 2016. https://theconversation.com/do-humans-need-dairy-heres-the-science-70434.

Mero A. Leucine supplementation and intensive training. Sports Med. 1999 Jun;27(6):347-58. doi: 10.2165/00007256-199927060-00001. PMID: 10418071.

Mobley CB, Haun CT, Roberson PA, et al. Effects of Whey, Soy or Leucine Supplementation with 12 Weeks of Resistance Training on Strength, Body Composition, and Skeletal Muscle and Adipose Tissue Histological Attributes in College-Aged Males. Nutrients. 2017;9(9):972. Published 2017 Sep 4. doi:10.3390/nu9090972

National Institutes of Health (NIH). Dietary Supplements for Exercise and Athletic Performance. Fact Sheet for Health Professionals. Updated on October 17, 2019. Retrieved from https://ods.od.nih.gov/factsheets/ExerciseAndAthleticPerformance-HealthProfessional/

National Institute on Alcohol Abuse and Alcoholism. "Alcohol's Effects on the Body." National Institutes of Health, October 2004. https://www.niaaa.nih.gov/alcohol-health/alcohols-effects-body.

National Research Council (US) Subcommittee on the Tenth Edition of the Recommended Dietary Allowances. Washington, DC: National Academies Press, 1989, 6, Protein and Amino Acids. https://www.ncbi.nlm.nih.gov/books/NBK234922/.

Neal, E. G., H. Chaffe, R. H. Schwartz, et al. "The Ketogenic Diet for the Treatment of Childhood Epilepsy: A Randomised Controlled Trial." *Lancet Neurology* 7, no. 6 (2008): 500–6.

https://doi.org/10.1016/S1474-4422(08)70092-9. Retrieved from https://www.ncbi.nlm.nih.gov/pubmed/18456557.

NIH, National Institute of General Medical Sciences. "The Biology of Fats in the Body." ScienceDaily, April 23, 2013. Accessed April 29, 2020. www.sciencedaily.com/releases/2013/04/130423102127.htm.

Norwitz, N. G., S. S. Dalai, and C. M. Palmer. "Ketogenic Diet as a Metabolic Treatment for Mental Illness." *Current Opinion Endocrinology, Diabetes, and Obesity* 5 (October 2020): 10. https://doi.org/10.1097/MED.0000000000000564.

Novin ZS, Ghavamzadeh S, Mehdizadeh A. The Weight Loss Effects of Branched Chain Amino Acids and Vitamin B6: A Randomized Controlled Trial on Obese and Overweight Women. Int J Vitam Nutr Res. 2018 Feb;88(1-2):80-89. doi: 10.1024/0300-9831/a000511. Epub 2019 Mar 6. PMID: 30841823.

O'Sullivan, Johnathan J. "The Science of Milk." TED talk. https://thekidshouldseethis.com/post/the-science-of-milk and https://www.youtube.com/watch?v=xmNzUEmFZMg.

Owen, O. E., A. P. Morgan, H. G. Kemp, J. M. Sullivan, M. G. Herrera, and G. F. Cahill Jr. "Brain Metabolism during Fasting." *Journal of Clinical Investigation* 46, no. 10 (1967): 1589–95. https://doi.org/10.1172/JCI105650. Retrieved from https://www.ncbi.nlm.nih.gov/pubmed/6061736/.

Owen, O. E., P. Felig, A. P. Morgan, J. Wahren, and G. F. Cahill Jr. "Liver and Kidney Metabolism during Prolonged Starvation." *Journal of Clinical Investigation* 48, no. 3 (1969): 574–83. https://doi.org/10.1172/JCI106016. Retrieved from https://www.ncbi.nlm.nih.gov/pubmed/5773093/.

Pacheco et al. "A Pilot Study of the Ketogenic Diet in Schizophrenia." *American Journal of Psychiatry* 121 (1965): 1110–11.

Palmer, Christopher, M. "Are Americans Addicted to Screens—or Just Burned Out?"

———. "Chronic Schizophrenia Put into Remission without Medication." April 6, 2019.

———. "Diabetes and Depression: Which Comes First?"

———. "Diets and Disorders: Can Foods or Fasting Be Considered Psychopharmacologic Therapies?" *Journal of Clinical Psychiatry* 81, no. 1 (July 9, 2018). https://doi.org/ 10.4088/ JCP.19ac12727.

———. "Don't Waste These Difficult Days."

———. "The Effects of the Ketogenic Diet on Psychiatric Symptomatology, Weight, and Metabolic Dysfunction in Schizophrenia Patients."

———. "Exercise and Fasting Linked to Brain Detox."

———. "Is It Safe to Face Your Trauma?"

———. "The Ketogenic Diet for Schizophrenia."

———. "The Ketogenic Diet in Medicine and Psychiatry."

———. "Ketogenic Diet in the Treatment of Schizoaffective Disorder: Two Case Studies." *Schizophrenia Research* 189 (November 2017): 208–09. https://doi.org/10.1016/j.schres.2017.01.053.

———. "The Ketogenic Diet May Help Stop Seizures." *Advancing Psychiatry*, March 26, 2019.

———. "Keto Nutrition from Science to Application," January 21, 2019.

———. "Making Sense of Nutritional Psychiatry."

———. "The Mental Health Survival Guide to the Pandemic: Threats."

———. "Six Steps to Stop an Addiction to Sugar and Junk Food."

Palmer, C. M., J. Gilbert-Jaramillo, and E. C. Westman. "The Ketogenic Diet and Remission of Psychotic Symptoms in Schizophrenia: Two Case Studies." *Schizophrenia Research* 208 (June 2019): 439–40. https://doi.org/10.1016/j.schres.2019.03.019.

Palsdottir, Hrefna. "What Is Ketosis, and Is It Healthy?" June 3, 2017. Healthline. https://www.healthline.com/nutrition/what-is-ketosis.

Paoli, A., A. Rubini, J. S. Volek, and K. A. Grimaldi. "Beyond Weight Loss: A Review of the Therapeutic Uses of Very-Low-Carbohydrate (Ketogenic) Diets" [published correction appears in *European Journal of Clinical Nutrition* 68, no. 5 (May 2014): 641]. *European Journal of Clinical Nutrition* 67, no. 8 (2013): 789–96. https://doi.org/10.1038/ejcn.2013.116. Retrieved from https://www.ncbi.nlm.nih.gov/pubmed/23801097/.

Paoli, A., K. Grimaldi, L. Toniolo, M. Canato, A. Bianco, and A. Fratter. "Nutrition and Acne: Therapeutic Potential of Ketogenic Diets." *Skin Pharmacology and Physiology* 25, no. 3 (2012): 111–17. https://doi.org/10.1159/000336404. Retrieved from https://www.ncbi.nlm.nih.gov/pubmed/22327146.

Parry SM, Puthucheary ZA. The impact of extended bed rest on the musculoskeletal system in the critical care environment. Extrem Physiol Med. 2015;4:16. Published 2015 Oct 9. doi:10.1186/s13728-015-0036-7

Pearson, Keith. "What Are the Key Functions of Carbohydrates?" Healthline, November 9, 2017. https://www.healthline.com/nutrition/carbohydrate-functions.

Pedroso JA, Zampieri TT, Donato J Jr. Reviewing the Effects of L-Leucine Supplementation in the Regulation of Food Intake, Energy Balance, and Glucose Homeostasis. Nutrients. 2015;7(5):3914-3937. Published 2015 May 22. doi:10.3390/nu7053914

Peterson, J. "The Scientifically Proven Natural Hangover Cure: Asparagus." Planet Green. Accessed September 5, 2017. http:// home.howstuffworks.com/green-living/scientists-asparagus-ward-hangover.htm.

Petre, Alina. "BCAA Benefits: A Review of Branched-Chain Amino Acids." Healthline, November 25, 2016. https://www. healthline.com/nutrition/bcaa.

Phelps et al. "The Ketogenic Diet for Type II Bipolar Disorder." *Neurocase* 19, no. 5 (2013): 423–26.

Picincu, Andra. "What Are Some Disadvantages of Dairy Milk?" LiveStrong, April 4, 2019. https://www.livestrong.com/ article/469499-what-are-some-disadvantages-of-milk/.

Qin LQ, Xun P, Bujnowski D, et al. Higher branched-chain amino acid intake is associated with a lower prevalence of being overweight or obese in middle-aged East Asian and Western adults. J Nutr. 2011;141(2):249-254. doi:10.3945/jn.110.128520

Rahimi MH, Shab-Bidar S, Mollahosseini M, Djafarian K. Branched-chain amino acid supplementation and exercise-induced muscle damage in exercise recovery: A meta-analysis of randomized clinical trials. Nutrition. 2017 Oct;42:30-36. doi: 10.1016/j.nut.2017.05.005. Epub 2017 May 18. Erratum in: Nutrition. 2017 Dec 22;: PMID: 28870476.

Rao TS, Asha MR, Ramesh BN, Rao KS. Understanding nutrition, depression and mental illnesses. Indian J Psychiatry. 2008;50(2):77-82. doi:10.4103/0019-5545.42391

Reinagel, Monica. "Is Drinking Milk Unnatural?" *Scientific American*, September 1, 2018. https://www.scientificamerican.com/ article/is-drinking-milk-unnatural/.

Ribeiro RV, Solon-Biet SM, Pulpitel T, et al. Of Older Mice and Men: Branched-Chain Amino Acids and Body Composition.

Nutrients. 2019;11(8):1882. Published 2019 Aug 13. doi:10.3390/nu11081882

Roberts, M. N., M. A. Wallace, A. A. Tomilov, et al. "A Ketogenic Diet Extends Longevity and Healthspan in Adult Mice." *Cell Metabolism* 26, no. 3 (September 5, 2017): 539–46.e5.

Rogers, A. "Everything Science Knows about Hangovers—and How to Cure Them." *Wired*, May 20, 2014. Retrieved from https://www.wired.com/2014/05/hangover-cure/

Roussell, Mike, and Lauren Mazzo. "Is Dairy Healthy? The Pros and Cons of Consuming Dairy." Shape.com. https://www.shape.com/healthy-eating/healthy-drinks/ask-diet-doctor-is-dairy-healthy.

Samaha, F. F., N. Iqbal, P. Seshadri, K. L. Chicano, D. A. Daily, J. McGrory, et al. "A Low-Carbohydrate as Compared with a Low-Fat Diet in Severe Obesity." *New England Journal of Medicine* 348, no. 21 (2003): 2074–81.

Sampath, A., E. H. Kossoff, S. L. Furth, P. L. Pyzik, and E. P. Vining. "Kidney Stones and the Ketogenic Diet: Risk Factors and Prevention." *Journal of Child Neurology* 22, no. 4 (2007): 375–78. https://doi.org/10.1177/0883073807301926. Retrieved from https://www.ncbi.nlm.nih.gov/pubmed/17621514.

Sapir, D. G., O. E. Owen, J. T. Cheng, R. Ginsberg, G. Boden, and W. G. Walker. "The Effect of Carbohydrates on Ammonium and Ketoacid Excretion during Starvation." *Journal of Clinical Investigation* 51, no. 8 (1972): 2093–2102. https://doi.org/10.1172/JCI107016. Retrieved from https://www.ncbi.nlm.nih.gov/pmc/articles/PMC292366/.

Sarnyai, Sarnyai, Z., A. K. Kraeuter, and C. M. Palmer. "Ketogenic Diet for Schizophrenia: Clinical Implication." *Current Opinions in Psychiatry* 32, no. 5 (September 2019): 394–401. https://doi.org/10.1097/YCO.0000000000000535.

Saslow, L., J. Daubenmier, J. Moskowitz, S. Kim, E. Murphy, S. Phinney, R. Ploutz-Snyder, V. Goldman, R. Cox, A. Mason, P. Moran, and F. Hecht. (2017). "Twelve-Month Outcomes of a Randomized Trial of a Moderate-Carbohydrate versus Very Low-Carbohydrate Diet in Overweight Adults with Type 2 Diabetes Mellitus or Prediabetes." *Nutrition & Diabetes* (December 21, 2017). https://www.nature.com/articles/s41387-017-0006-9.

Schmitt, Barton D. *Cow's Milk: Pros and Cons.* Summit Medical Group, 2014. https://www.summitmedicalgroup.com/library/pediatric_health/hhg_cows_milk/.

Sharman, M. J., W. J. Kraemer, D. M. Love, et al. "A Ketogenic Diet Favorably Affects Serum Biomarkers for Cardiovascular Disease in Normal-Weight Men." *Journal of Nutrition* 132, no. 7 (2002):1879–85. https://doi.org/10.1093/jn/132.7.1879. Retrieved from https://www.ncbi.nlm.nih.gov/pubmed/12097663/.

Simonson M, Boirie Y, Guillet C. Protein, amino acids and obesity treatment. Rev Endocr Metab Disord. 2020;21(3):341-353. doi:10.1007/s11154-020-09574-5

Sirtoli, Raphael. "Snack Nation: 121 Easy and Delicious Healthy Snacks in 2020 for Every Type of Snacker." Snack Safely. https://snacksafely.com/safe-snack-guide/.

Snorgaard, O., G. M. Poulsen, H. K. Andersen, et al. "Systematic Review and Meta-Analysis of Dietary Carbohydrate Restriction in Patients with Type 2 Diabetes." *BMJ Open Diabetes Research and Care* 5, no. 1 (2017). https://doi.org/10.1136/bmjdrc-2016-000354.

Sohn, Emily. "Drinking Milk: The Pros and Cons." *Los Angeles Times,* March 20, 2015. https://www.latimes.com/health/la-he-milk-20150321-story.html.

"Sprite May Be the Best Hangover Cure, Chinese Researchers Say." *Huffington Post*, October 9, 2013. http://www.huffingtonpost.com/2013/10/09/sprite-hangover-cure_n_4071282.html.

Steen, Juliette. "A Simple Guide to Healthy Snacking: There's Only Four Basic Things to Remember." *Huffington Post*, March 23, 2017. https://www.huffingtonpost.com.au/2017/03/22/a-simple-guide-to-healthy-snacking_a_21904746/.

Stern, L., N. Iqbal, P. Seshadri, et al. "The Effects of Low-Carbohydrate versus Conventional Weight Loss Diets in Severely Obese Adults: One-Year Follow-Up of a Randomized Trial." *Annals of Internal Medicine* 140, no. 10 (2004): 778–85. https://doi.org/10.7326/0003-4819-140-10-200405180-00007. Retrieved from https://www.ncbi.nlm.nih.gov/pubmed/15148064.

Stevenson, Sarah. "10 Healthier Sugar Alternatives You Should Try." *Senior Living Blog: A Place for Mom*, February 17, 2015. https://www.aplaceformom.com/blog/2-17-15-healthy-sugar-alternatives/.

Suares, N. C., and A. C. Ford. "Systematic Review: The Effects of Fibre in the Management of Chronic Idiopathic Constipation." *Alimentary Pharmacology & Therapeutics* 33, no. 8 (2011): 895–901. https://doi.org/10.1111/j.1365-2036.2011.04602.x. Retrieved from https://pubmed.ncbi.nlm.nih.gov/21332763/.

Tanja Kongerslev, Anne Raben, Tine Tholstrup, Sabita S. Soedamah-Muthu, Ian Givens, and Arne Astrup. "Milk and Dairy Products: Good or Bad for Human Health? An Assessment of the Totality of Scientific Evidence." *Food & Nutrition Research* 60 (November 22, 2016). https://doi.org/10.3402/fnr.v60.32527. Retrieved from https://www.ncbi.nlm.nih.gov/pmc/articles/PMC5122229/.

Thorning, Tobias, K. Deirdre, et al. "Effect of Low-Fat Diet Interventions versus Other Diet Interventions on Long-Term Weight Change in Adults: A Systematic Review and

Meta-Analysis." *Lancet Diabetes & Endocrinology* 3, no. 12 (2015): 968–79.

"Top 10 Pro and Con Arguments: Is Drinking Milk Healthy for Humans?" https://milk.procon.org/top-10-pro-con-arguments/.

Tosh, S. M. "Review of Human Studies Investigating the Post-Prandial Blood-Glucose-Lowering Ability of Oat and Barley Food Products." *European Journal of Clinical Nutrition* 67, no. 4 (April 2013): 310–17. https://doi.org/10.1038/ejcn.2013.25. Retrieved from https://pubmed.ncbi.nlm.nih.gov/23422921/.

"The Truth about Alcohol." Foundation for a Drug-Free World. http://www.drugfreeworld.org/drugfacts/alcohol/short-term-long-term-effects.html.

"The Truth about What Alcohol Does to Your Body." QuitAlcohol. https://www.quitalcohol.com/the-truth-about-what-alcohol-does-to-your-body.html.

University of North Carolina. "What's the Best Hangover Cure?" *Medical News Today*, December 4, 2015. http://www.medicalnewstoday.com/articles/173349.php.

Valerio A, D'Antona G, Nisoli E. Branched-chain amino acids, mitochondrial biogenesis, and healthspan: an evolutionary perspective. Aging (Albany NY). 2011;3(5):464-478. doi:10.18632/aging.100322

Van De Wall, MS, RD, Gavin. 5 Proven Benefits of BCAAs (Branched-Chain Amino Acids). Healthline, July 11, 2018. Retrieved from https://www.healthline.com/nutrition/benefits-of-bcaa#TOC_TITLE_HDR_2

VanDusseldorp TA, Escobar KA, Johnson KE, et al. Effect of Branched-Chain Amino Acid Supplementation on Recovery Following Acute Eccentric Exercise. Nutrients. 2018;10(10):1389. Published 2018 Oct 1. doi:10.3390/nu10101389

Van Walleghen EL, Orr JS, Gentile CL, Davy BM. Pre-meal water consumption reduces meal energy intake in older but not younger subjects. Obesity (Silver Spring). 2007;15(1):93-99. doi:10.1038/oby.2007.506. Retrieved from https://www.ncbi.nlm.nih.gov/pubmed/17228036

Van Walleghen EL, Orr JS, Gentile CL, Davy BM. Pre-meal water consumption reduces meal energy intake in older but not younger subjects. Obesity (Silver Spring). 2007;15(1):93-99. doi:10.1038/oby.2007.506. Retrieved from https://www.ncbi.nlm.nih.gov/pubmed/17228036

Vanitallie, T. B., C. Nonas, A. Di Rocco, K. Boyar, K. Hyams, and S. B. Heymsfield. "Treatment of Parkinson Disease with Diet-Induced Hyperketonemia: A Feasibility Study." *Neurology* 64, no. 4 (2005): 728–30. https://doi.org/10.1212/01.WNL.0000152046.11390.45. Retrieved from https://www.ncbi.nlm.nih.gov/pubmed/15728303/.

Volek, J. S., M. J. Sharman, and C. E. Forsythe. "Modification of Lipoproteins by Very Low-Carbohydrate Diets." *Journal of Nutrition* 135, no. 6 (2005): 1339–42. https://doi.org/10.1093/jn/135.6.1339. Retrieved from https://www.ncbi.nlm.nih.gov/pubmed/15930434/.

Volek, J., M. Sharman, A. Gómez, et al. "Comparison of Energy-Restricted Very Low-Carbohydrate and Low-Fat Diets on Weight Loss and Body Composition in Overweight Men and Women." *Nutrition & Metabolism* (London) 1, no. 1 (November 8, 2004): 13. https://www.ncbi.nlm.nih.gov/pubmed/15533250/.

Waldron M, Whelan K, Jeffries O, Burt D, Howe L, Patterson SD. The effects of acute branched-chain amino acid supplementation on recovery from a single bout of hypertrophy exercise in resistance-trained athletes. Appl Physiol Nutr Metab. 2017 Jun;42(6):630-636. doi: 10.1139/apnm-2016-0569. Epub 2017 Jan 27. PMID: 28177706.

Warwick, Kathy. "13 Legitimate Ways to Stop a Hangover." The Greatist. https://greatist.com/health/13-legit-ways-stop-hangover.

Weintraub, Karen. "Prescription: More Broccoli, Fewer Carbs—How Some Doctors Are Looking to Food to Treat Illness." WBUR, an NPR station, June 4, 2019.

Westman, E. C., W.-S. Yancy Jr., J. C. Mavropoulos, M. Marquart, and J. R. McDuffie. "The Effect of a Low-Carbohydrate, Ketogenic Diet versus a Low-Glycemic Index Diet on Glycemic Control in Type 2 Diabetes Mellitus." *Nutrition & Metabolism* (London) 5 (December 19, 2008): 36. https://doi.org/10.1186/1743-7075-5-36. Retrieved from https://www.ncbi.nlm.nih.gov/pubmed/19099589/.

Whitmore, Lisa. "Our Game-Changing Guide to Healthy Snacking." Real Simple. Updated August 2, 2019. https://www.realsimple.com/health/nutrition-diet/healthy-eating/healthy-snacking.

Wibisono, C., N. Rowe, E. Beavis, et al. "Ten-Year Single-Center Experience of the Ketogenic Diet: Factors Influencing Efficacy, Tolerability, and Compliance." *Journal of Pediatrics* 166, no. 4 (2015): 1030–36.e1. https://doi.org/10.1016/j.jpeds.2014.12.018. Retrieved from https://www.ncbi.nlm.nih.gov/pubmed/25649120.

Włodarczyk, Adam, Mariusz S. Wiglusz, and Wiesław Jerzy Cubała. "Ketogenic Diet for Schizophrenia: Nutritional Approach to Antipsychotic Treatment." *Medical Hypotheses* 118 (September 2018): 74–77. https://doi.org/10.1016/j.mehy.2018.06.022.

Wu, P. Y., J. Edmond, N. Auestad, S. Rambathla, J. Benson, and T. Picone. "Medium-Chain Triglycerides in Infant Formulas and Their Relation to Plasma Ketone Body Concentrations." *Pediatric Research* 20, no. 4 (1986): 338–41. https://doi.org/10.1203/00006450-198604000-00016. Retrieved from https://www.ncbi.nlm.nih.gov/pubmed/3703623.

Yancy, W. S. Jr., M. K. Olsen, J. R. Guyton, R. P. Bakst, and E. C. Westman. "A Low-Carbohydrate, Ketogenic Diet versus a Low-Fat Diet to Treat Obesity and Hyperlipidemia: A Randomized, Controlled Trial." *Annals of Internal Medicine* 140, no. 10 (2004): 769–77. https://doi.org/10.7326/0003-4819-140-10-200405180-00006. Retrieved from https://www.ncbi.nlm.nih.gov/pubmed/15148063.

Yaroslovsky et al. "Ketogenic Diet in Bipolar Illness." *Bipolar Disorders* 4 (2002): 75.

Zamani, G. R., M. Mohammadi, M. R. Ashrafi, et al. "The Effects of Classic Ketogenic Diet on Serum Lipid Profile in Children with Refractory Seizures." *Acta Neurologica Belgica* 116, no. 4 (2016): 529–34. https://doi.org/10.1007/s13760-016-0601-x. Retrieved from https://www.ncbi.nlm.nih.gov/pubmed/26791878.

Zhou, W., P. Mukherjee, M. A. Kiebish, W. T. Markis, J. G. Mantis, and T. N. Seyfried. "The Calorically Restricted Ketogenic Diet, an Effective Alternative Therapy for Malignant Brain Cancer." *Nutrition & Metabolism* (London) 4 (February 21, 2007): 5. https://doi.org/10.1186/1743-7075-4-5. Retrieved from https://www.ncbi.nlm.nih.gov/pubmed/17313687/.

Zoltán, and Christopher M. Palmer. "Ketogenic Therapy in Serious Mental Illness: Emerging Evidence." *International Journal of Neuropsychopharmacology* 23, no. 7 (July 2020): 434–39. https://doi.org/10.1093/ijnp/pyaa036.

INDEX OF RESEARCH STUDIES, CASE REPORTS, CLINICAL TRIALS, ARTICLES, AUTHORS, AND EXPERTS

INDEX

About The NUTRIENT Diet

Since the 1980s I've literally observed hundreds of diet plans come and go—although, a few of them, like Weight Watchers®, Jenny Craig®, Slim Fast® and Nutrisystem®, have appeared to stand the tests of time. However, most of them, seem to come and go like the wind. And, I got to see this up close and personal within my own family, within myself and within the clients of my practices. Through all of these observations, and taking an analytic approach to them both singularly and in aggregate, I came to the conclusion that the vast majority of diet plans and approaches "FAIL" because they expect the individual to make too many primary changes at once. In essence, they expect you to change overnight (instead of doing so gradually and naturally), leading most dieters feeling frustrated and overwhelmed. And, plans, goals and objectives tend to fail when they require too many steps too quickly. I base this opinion off of the "Simplicity Principle", which I state as 'the simpler something is to set up and begin, the more likely one is to consistently continue (i.e., perpetuate) it.' The reverse of that is the "Complexity Principle", which I state as 'the more complicated something is to set up, begin and/or perpetuate, then the more likely one is to abruptly discontinue (i.e., abandon) it eventually.' The same is true of most diets (i.e., lifestyle modification plans [LMPs]). Because they are generally complex (and unpleasant), even when someone strives to make them easy, they are difficult to permanently install as a habit, routine &/or ritual. That's WHY it's so difficult for the vast majority of individuals to start, continue and complete a diet (or other lifestyle plan); and to continue to maintain the habits required to keep their new weight.

The Nutrient Diet is a completely new, bold, intelligent, modern, psychological approach to diet, health, wellness and weight management habits! The Nutrient Diet is a "Lifestyle Approach" for general & mental health based on sound psychological principles! The Nutrient Diet is 50% Diet and Nutrition, and 50% Cognitive and Behavioral Psychological Strategies for eating behaviors, dieting, impulse control and habit formation. The Nutrient Diet is the first book of its kind to take a "Cognitive Behavioral" (i.e., Psychological) approach to diet, nutrition, health, wellness, weight loss, weight management and lifestyle management! The Nutrient Diet truly is a "Trendsetter" in the diet, health, wellness, medicine, nutrition, weight loss, weight management and lifestyle fields! Not only does The Nutrient Diet show and explain WHAT you need to eat, The Nutrient Diet explains HOW & WHY you should eat it—based on sound, tested scientific data, clinical trials and psychological principles! The Nutrient Diet does so in a way that teaches and coaches you to make lifestyle changes easily, naturally, gradually and progressively so that you don't get frustrated and overwhelmed along the way... Even more, The Nutrient Diet augments other dietary plans (Like Nutrisystem®, Weight Watchers®, Slim Fast® and Jenny Craig®) with nutritional facts, concepts, principles and explanations in a straightforward way that makes it much less likely that you'll fail or abandon them. So, The Nutrient Diet will help you even if you're already using another dietary plan! The Nutrient Diet plays well with others! The Nutrient Diet is a must read for anyone interested in creating and maintaining good health and managing their weight without dreading it!

David A. Wright, MD, MM, MBA, MHSA (Dr. David)

Dr. Wright's new lifestyle, health, wellness, weight loss, nutrition & diet book, The Nutrient Diet, could not have come at a better time in history. Nutrition and diet are the building blocks of all metabolic activity, and they form the underpinnings of both general and mental health. I have been using ketogenic diets to treat patients with psychiatric disorders ranging from major depressive disorder to bipolar disorder to schizophrenia for almost two decades. As such, I understand all too well just how crucial nutrition and diet are to general health, neural health and mental health. By presenting a succinct book that combines all of the central medical concepts of nutrition with psychological strategies for maintaining a host of new dietary, wellness, health, weight management and lifestyle choices & behaviors, Dr. Wright has found a unique, logical, and flexible method of answering the three most crucial questions when it comes to diet, nutrition, health, wellness, weight and mental health: (1) "what should I eat" (2) "how should I eat it" (3) "why should I eat it"; in a single book!

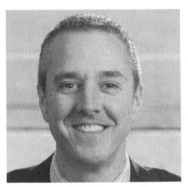

Christopher M. Palmer, MD, Board Certified Psychiatrist, Harvard Psychiatric Expert on The Ketogenic Diet

This lifestyle, health, wellness, weight loss, nutrition & diet book could not be conceived and written at a more prescient time than during a pandemic that stresses even the most hearty and stable among us. It is well known in the field of mental health that what we ingest has a direct and observable effect on our psychological wellbeing and functioning. The building blocks of all essential neurotransmitters are vitamins, minerals and amino acids that are found in sensible and healthy meal plans; but often we, as individuals, and as a society, make accomplishing this more complicated than it needs to be. Dr. Wright's book herein brilliantly breaks down the roadmap to success in both being and eating healthy to a few simple and easily achievable steps attainable in a reasonable time frame. The Nutrient Diet is a must read for anyone who wishes to take a more holistic approach to better living and improved satisfaction with their daily lives and mental functioning.

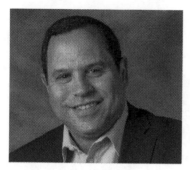

Todd M. Antin, MD, Board Certified in Adult, Addiction, Forensic & Geriatric Psychiatry Emory Quadruple Board Certified Expert in Psychiatry

For those who wish to maintain or improve their health by eating properly, Dr. Wright's book *The Nutrient Diet*, informative and inspirational from a medical clinician's perspective, is an excellent place to start. From a biblical perspective, Genesis 9:3 says, "Everything that lives and moves will be food for you. Just as I gave you the green plants, I now give you everything." This statement is self-explanatory. However, additional warnings are found in Proverbs 23:20–21. These verses warn us not to be gluttonous in our consumption of food or drink. Dr. Wright splendidly reminds us that we are what we eat and that all dietary consumption should be done in moderation. In just twelve short weeks, by following Dr. Wright's instructions, starting with a balanced consumption of water and ending with bonus general health and mental health nuggets, you will be able to bring your life to a state of both physical and mental health excellence. I thank God for blessing us with someone (who happens to be my son) who wrote such an enlightening book.

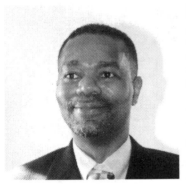

Pastor Harlis R. Wright, Master of Science, Biology; Master of Divinity, Columbia Theological Seminary Pastor, Faith Presbyterian Church (Pine Bluff, Arkansas) Science professor, thirty-five years

About Dr. David

Dr. David A. Wright achieved his MD in July of 2010, graduating Suma Cum Laude [4.0 GPA] from Xavier University School of Medicine. His primary emphases in medical school were forensic psychiatry, addiction psychiatry (addiction medicine), and neurology. While attending medical school, Dr. Wright concurrently completed 3 Masters degrees back to back: an MHSA in healthcare law and policy, an MBA in healthcare administration and an MM in healthcare management.

After completing his MD and three Masters degrees, Dr. Wright became a Forensic Psychiatric Consultant for the largest psychiatric practice in the southeastern United States, PACT Atlanta (since 2010). Instead of pursing a residency in psychiatry Dr. Wright chose to study and train in disciplines that were more in line with the techniques used by the Father and Uncle of Psychiatry, Dr. Sigmund Freud (The Father of Psychiatry) and Dr. Milton Erickson (The Uncle of Psychiatry), respectively. As such, he chose to approach mental health from a more natural, holistic, root cause-based, logic-centered and analytical outlook instead of choosing an approach primarily based on handing out pills to simply address the surface symptoms rather than addressing the underlying, root causes (which is how psychiatry is generally practiced today). Dr. Wright believes that society needs more real solutions, not more pills. Finally, in 2016, Dr. Wright completed his formal training in those disciplines and opened his first practice, MLC Of Greater Atlanta, in Decatur, Georgia, across the street from Emory DeKalb Medical Center. Dr. Wright opened his 2nd practice, Atlanta Coaching & Hypnotherapy Associates (Also Known as Atlanta Coaching), in 2018.

Website Info: www.mlcoga.com
www.atlantacoaching.com

Dr. David A. Wright is the clinical director of MLC of Greater Atlanta [MLCOGA] and Atlanta Coaching & Hypnotherapy Associates [ACHA]. MLC of Greater Atlanta specializes in helping clients who have been diagnosed with the following disorders and conditions, among others: anxiety disorders, adjustment disorders, grief, stress disorders, obsessive compulsive disorder, sleep disorders, panic disorders, phobias, mood disorders, mild to moderate depression, ADD/ADHD, PTSD, personality disorders, learning disabilities, and childhood and adolescent behavioral issues without the use of medications or psychiatric pharmaceutical agents. MLC of Greater Atlanta specializes in helping clients who desire to lose weight, quit smoking, drop destructive habits, change life direction, improve relationships, achieve success and make permanent, long-lasting positive life changes. Atlanta Coaching & Hypnotherapy Associates is primarily focused on providing hypnosis and hypnotherapy.

Dr. Wright is a Physician (i.e., an M.D.), a Board Certified Hypnotherapist, a Board Certified NLP Practitioner, a Board Certified Coach, & a Board Certified Time Line Therapy ® Practitioner who specializes in Non-Pharmacologic, root cause-based, logic-centered, psychoanalytic methods of helping individuals and groups to achieve positive changes and breakthroughs. Dr. Wright is presently accepting new clients and referrals. Dr. Wright also provides consulting services to other healthcare professionals and is a featured speaker and corporate trainer. He is an expert in the areas of "Change Management", "Personal & Professional Development" and "Performance Improvement."

Dr. Wright's current and upcoming books include (1) Sweet Potato Pie for the Spirit, Soul & Psyche (a self-improvement & self-empowerment book) (2) Tomato Bisque for the Brain (a self-improvement & self-empowerment book) (3) The Nutrient Diet (a diet, nutrition, health, wellness, weight loss, weight management and lifestyle management book based on "Cognitive Behavioral" approaches and the psychology of habit formation) (4) The Universal Secrets (a self-improvement & self-empowerment book) (5) Alternative, Holistic & Psychoanalytic Mental Health Approaches (a book for those seeking therapies and life solutions without the use of psychotropic medications). Dr. Wright also has additonal books in progress on a variety of subjects and topics.

DIET/NUTRITION/WEIGHT LOSS/EATING/HEALTH/WELLNESS/FITNESS

The vast majority of dietary plans and approaches "FAIL" because they expect the individual to make too many primary changes too quickly. In essence, they expect you to change overnight (instead of doing so gradually and naturally), leading most dieters feeling frustrated and overwhelmed.

The NUTRIENT Diet is a completely new, bold, modern psychological approach to diet, health, wellness and weight management habits. The NUTRIENT Diet is a "Lifestyle Approach" to general & mental health based on sound psychological principles. The NUTRIENT Diet is 50% Diet and Nutrition, and 50% Cognitive and Behavioral Psychological Strategies for eating behaviors, dieting, impulse control and habit formation. The NUTRIENT Diet is the first book of its kind to take a "Cognitive Behavioral" (i.e., Psychological) approach to diet, nutrition, health, wellness, weight loss, weight management and lifestyle management! The NUTRIENT Diet not only shows and explains WHAT, HOW & WHY you should eat certain foods based on sound, tested scientific data, clinical trials and psychological principles. It teaches and coaches you to make lifestyle changes easily, naturally, gradually and progressively so that you don't get overwhelmed… Even more, The NUTRIENT Diet augments other dietary plans (Like Nutrisystem ®, Weight Watchers ®, Slim Fast ®, Jenny Craig ®, etc.) with nutritional facts, concepts, principles and explanations in a straightforward way that makes it less likely that you'll fail or abandon them. So, The NUTRIENT Diet will help you even if you're already using another diet plan! The NUTRIENT Diet plays well with others!

—David A. Wright, MD, MM, MBA, MHSA

I have been using ketogenic diets to treat patients for almost two decades. I understand all too well just how crucial nutrition and diet are to general health, neural health and mental health. By combining all of the central medical concepts of nutrition with psychological strategies for maintaining health and lifestyle choices and behaviors, Dr. Wright has created a unique, logical, and flexible method of answering the three most crucial questions when it comes to diet, nutrition, health, wellness and weight: (1) "what should I eat" (2) "how should I eat it" (3) "why should I eat it"; in a single book!

—Christopher M. Palmer, MD, Board Certified Psychiatrist, Harvard Psychiatric Expert on The Ketogenic Diet

This lifestyle, health, wellness, weight loss, nutrition & diet book could not be conceived and written at a more prescient time than during a pandemic. Dr. Wright's book brilliantly breaks down the roadmap to success in both being and eating healthy to a few simple and easily achievable steps attainable in a reasonable time frame.

—Todd M. Antin, MD, Board Certified in Adult, Addiction, Forensic & Geriatric Psychiatry Emory Quadruple Board Certified Expert in Psychiatry

Website Info: www.mlcoga.com
www.atlantacoaching.com

Dr. David A. Wright achieved his MD in July of 2010, graduating Suma Cum Laude [4.0 GPA] from Xavier University School of Medicine. While attending medical school, Dr. Wright concurrently completed 3 Masters degrees back to back: an MHSA in healthcare law and policy, an MBA in healthcare administration and an MM in healthcare management. Instead of pursing a residency in psychiatry Dr. Wright chose to study and train in disciplines that were more natural, holistic, root cause-based, logic-centered and analytical in their approach instead of choosing an approach primarily based on handing out pills to simply address the surface symptoms rather than addressing the underlying, root causes (which is how psychiatry is generally practiced today). Dr. Wright believes that society needs more real solutions, not more pills. Dr. David A. Wright is the clinical director of MLC of Greater Atlanta [MLCOGA] and Atlanta Coaching & Hypnotherapy Associates [ACHA]. MLC of Greater Atlanta specializes in helping clients who have been diagnosed with a number of psychological disorders and conditions without the use of medications or psychiatric pharmaceutical agents. His practices also specialize in helping clients who desire to lose weight, quit smoking, drop destructive habits, change life direction, improve relationships, achieve success and make permanent, long-lasting positive life changes.

Dr. Wright is a Physician (i.e., an M.D.), a Board Certified Hypnotherapist, a Board Certified NLP Practitioner, a Board Certified Coach, & a Board Certified Time Line Therapy ® Practitioner who specializes in non-pharmacologic, root cause-based, logic-centered psychoanalytic methods of helping individuals and groups to achieve positive changes and breakthroughs. Dr. Wright is an expert in the areas of "Change Management", "Personal & Professional Development" and "Performance Improvement."

U.S. $XX.XX

ISBN 978-1-6632-1017-3

90000

9 781663 210173

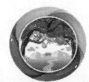

iUniverse ®
www.iuniverse.com

Printed in the United States
by Baker & Taylor Publisher Services